*The
Woman's
Total
Reshape
Program*

The Woman's Total Reshape Program

BY VERA ABRIEL

E. P. DUTTON / New York

For information contact: Elsevier-Dutton Publishing Co., Inc.,
2 Park Avenue, New York, N.Y. 10016

Library of Congress Cataloging in Publication Data

Abriel, Vera.
　The woman's total reshape program.
　1. Reducing exercises.　2. Exercise for women.　3. Reducing diets.　4. Adipose tissues.　I. Title.
RA781.6.A27　1980　613.7'1　80-185

ISBN: 0-525-93148-1

Published simultaneously in Canada by Clarke, Irwin & Company Limited, Toronto and Vancouver

10 9 8 7 6 5 4 3 2 1

FIRST EDITION

Contents

Introduction

When I first saw Vera Abriel's manuscript, I was amazed at how obvious the ideas seemed, and yet no one had put it all together into an entire program so comprehensively before! Here were the time-honored figure-shaping devices used by many of the luxury beauty-spas around the country—diet, exercise, massage, sauna, slanting board to counteract gravity, and others—all integrated into an easy program any woman can follow in the privacy of her home, without spending any money, or buying anything special—and it was safe and healthy, and it seemed like fun!

But this was not all. As I read on, I soon realized that this program was something special, entirely original. For in the Woman's Total Reshape Program, the familiar figure-control devices are organized in a new, scientifically co-ordinated way to make each component work twice as effectively, and with some results one would previously only dream about! In my years of involvement in the world of beauty and diet, exercise, rejuvenation, and health, both as an editor and as a writer, I had rarely come across a program that could do such wonderful things for a woman's figure!

I've been pleased and proud to be Vera Abriel's editor, and I hope that *The Woman's Total Reshape Program* brings you the figure you have always wanted—and should have.

Constance Schrader

AUTHOR OF:

WRINKLES: *How to Erase Them*

MAKEOVERS: *A Total New Image*

NINE TO FIVE: *Looks, Clothes, Personality*

A big thank you

To the thirty-six wonderful women—co-creators of the
Reshape Program—for their patience, ingenuity, and
determination; to the long-suffering librarians and
other custodians of information for unearthing for us
the latest in science and the earliest in "folk"
methods; and to the doctors of medicine,
nutritionists, and other experts for their professional
guidance and their understanding that a beautiful
body is a "privilege of nature" to which we should all
have an equal right.

PART I

The Woman's Total Reshape Program

ITS HISTORY,
ITS TRACK RECORD,
AND THE SCIENCE
BEHIND THE MAGIC.

1

Can a Woman Actually Change Her Figure?

Even in figure-shaping, men have it easier. We've all seen pictures of the former 130-pound weakling who's managed to weight-lift his puny frame to Mr. Universe proportions. But let a woman be unhappy with her wide hips, for instance, or with the relative smallness of her breasts, and she'll be told: "Forget it, dear. It's your heredity."

As a writer on nutrition, I had been studying the human body and what can be done with it for years, and my research into the findings of figure-control experts seemed to confirm this negative attitude. You can *lose* weight, they tell you (and if you succeed, which is often impermanent, your neck is likely to get thin and scrawny, your cheeks hollow, and your bust, if small to begin with, will practically disappear). Or you can *gain* weight on your bust (but then your hips and thighs will balloon out of all proportions), and you can tone your muscles. But up until now, to really *change* your figure the way a man can change his has been nothing but a dream.

Why the discrimination? Experts tell us it has to do with "android" (typically masculine) and "gynoid" (typically feminine) figure types.

Male and Female, There's a Difference!

Three major anatomical traits are said to contrast the gynoid type to the android type:

1. Gynoid adipose tissue (as *fat* is called) is three times larger than the android type.
2. Consequently, its fat/muscle ratio is on the average three times greater than for the android adipose tissue.
3. Gynoid adipose tissue develops mostly over the lower half of the body.

Of course, by gynoid and android types it isn't suggested that *all* women have gynoid nor that all men have android figure characteristics. What is meant is that the majority of women have large hips and thighs and smaller upper bodies, and therefore that is the gynoid type, while the majority of men have more muscle and less fat, and therefore that is the android type.

The "Ideal" vs. the "Typical"

Throughout the ages the tough, muscular male has always been both the "ideal" and the "typical" prototype. Not so for the female. True, there have been times when the "ideal" and the "typical" female shapes happily coincided: see the voluptuous Rubens ladies with their huge, undulating buttocks and dainty breasts. But that kind of beauty will not do for the modern woman. We want boyish hips and slim, taut bodies to go with our active lifestyle, and for femininity, we want well-developed breasts.

The Problem is Fat

Exercise will tighten or tone our muscles, but our principal concern is not muscle, but *fat*—too much of it in the wrong places. Through dieting we can lose weight, but we generally put it back on again, faster than we ever took it off in the first place! And we lose weight from the head down: first in the face, the neck, and the breasts—by the time we get to the hips and thighs, where most of our troubles lie, our upper bodies have all but wasted away. And even then, those ugly bulges on hips, thighs, and buttocks are often impossible to get rid of.

Why the stubbornness? It's because of the way our fat cells were laid down.

Can We Conquer Heredity?

Recent findings seem to indicate that the total number of fat cells we will have were laid down during our childhood and adolescence, following a pattern dictated by heredity. The pattern is often uneven, consisting of more densely laid down cells in some parts of the body than in others, and when all the cells are filled to capacity with fat, the areas of greater cell density will bulge, while the other areas will remain relatively lean. Supporting this theory is the fact that when certain kinds of laboratory rats have a section of their fat surgically removed, new fat cells to compensate for the missing sections will form only during their youthful, proliferating periods, but not thereafter. This being so, the experts are right: We adult women cannot hope to increase the numbers of our fat cells in any particular area, nor can we decrease them (an important argument against overfeeding our babies till they're "cute and chubby"!), yet we *can* vastly change our figures as the Reshape Method will show you. How? We can alter our shapes most effectively, not by increasing or decreasing the *number* of our fat cells in particular areas, but by altering their *size*. An empty fat cell is a *flat* cell, and it hardly matters how many there are in an area, while even a relatively few plump ones will add lovely feminine curves to your contours. The trick is to control where you want to keep them lean and where you want them to gorge themselves to several times their former size.

So if men can change their shapes, *we can*. The odds in the past may have been against us, but this will not be the first time that we women have proved "anything they can do . . ."

Let the experience of thirty-seven Aussie women show you how you can actually conquer heredity, and slim, trim, mold, and fill out your body to the fabulous proportions you always dreamed of but thought you could never have.

2

How Thirty-seven Australian Women Changed from Fat—or Flat—to Fabulous!

Originally, there were sixteen of us meeting for a eurhythmics class ("giggle and wiggle," we called it) in my home in Bellevue Hill, a Sydney Harbor suburb, every Friday morning. Though we differed in other aspects, all of us had two things in common: We all had figure problems with their attendant miseries, such as lack of self-confidence, avoidance of the beach (in surf-mad Sydney no less!), career obstacles (young Sheree dreamed of becoming a model, Patricia wanted to be an air hostess), impaired health (Paula had high blood pressure, while Leanne's circulatory problems originated in obesity), and, of course, setbacks to romance (Susanne, whose vital statistics were 32-27-41, imagined that she was losing her fiancé to his secretary, whose measurements were practically identical to her own, but *in reverse!*)—and we all loved to eat.

Maybe you feel that I should have said, "We all had figure problems *because* we liked to eat," but this is not necessarily so. In fact, although quite a few of us were just plain fat, there were many who suffered mainly from ugly flab on hips and thighs, or from spare tires around waist and midriff, and had always had those figure characteristics, even before our love of good food had made us put on extra pounds. And there were quite a few

7

who, though normal or overweight in the lower regions, were downright skinny from the waist up. If only one could grab a few inches *away* from hips and thighs, and *add them to the breasts!*

A Lesson from History

Helen was a fashion designer with a favorite theory. Every now and again she would point out that throughout history the nude female form had been made to conform to some external requirements—often not intentionally, but as a result of certain practices inspired by fashion, custom, or necessity. In the days of the crinoline or the bustle, for instance, when women's waists were tightly laced into tiny bodices but their lower bodies were free to sprawl under the huge camouflaging skirts, their hips and thighs and their half-exposed bosoms generally became voluptuous, while their waists became impossibly slim. Few of our slimmest models today could fit their waists into the "hourglass" bodices worn by an ordinary girl in Great-grandmother's day. On the other hand, some decades later, special brassieres and bust confiners of the flat-chested "flapper" era often had permanently flattening results.

One day Judy, whose divorce had just become final, complained that she had to get a jeweler to file through her wedding ring: After fourteen years of marriage and twenty pounds of weight-gain, she had not been able to get it off her finger.

She showed us her hand, and at that moment the Woman's Reshape Method was born. Though her wrist, the back of her hand, and her fingers were well padded with fat, the narrow band around her ring finger where the wedding ring had exerted pressure over the years was lean—you could actually feel the bone! At the same time, the rest of Judy's ring finger seemed distinctly fatter than the other fingers or the corresponding finger on her other hand, as if the ring had not only prevented fat from settling, but had shifted it to the surrounding areas.

An Experiment In Vivo

Many scientific experiments, as we subsequently learned, are carried out *in vitro*, meaning "in the glass" or test tube. Far fewer are conducted *in vivo*—on the live organism; and fewer still on the human being. Our experiments, which lasted a little over three years and resulted in a more than 90 percent success rate (I'll give results in the following text), were conducted on a group of very much alive and painfully human organisms who, being both the experimenters and the experimentees, were in a unique position to make our dream come true.

Throughout our experimentations, we consulted doctors, nutritionists, beauty experts, yoga teachers, pharmacists, and body builders. Four in our group were married to medical men, three had science degrees of their own. Marge's husband was a biochemist and she herself worked as a lab technician in the hematology department of Sydney's Prince Henry Hospital. In our final group—two of the original sixteen dropped out but others came, and eventually we numbered thirty-seven, varying in age from teen-age daughters of older members to two grandmothers over sixty—there was also one nutritionist and one physical education teacher who had spent half of her working life licking into shape flabby rich women in one of Europe's most celebrated health-and-beauty spas! The rest of us were businesswomen, homemakers, students, secretaries, but we all contributed something of importance: We all did research, and we all served as guinea pigs, sometimes as true subjects, at other times as controls.

Our goal was revolutionary, fantastic, and simple: to take whatever shapes nature and our indulgences had given us, and shape them—as quickly, effortlessly, and pleasantly as possible—into absolutely stunning proportions.

3

Our First Breakthrough

The first important breakthrough in our thinking occurred when we agreed on these points:

1. Though bone and muscle structures play important parts, the crucial aspect of figure beauty in women is *quantity and distribution of fat*.
2. Contrary to popular belief, even the breasts rely on *fat* rather than on glandular tissue for their size and shape.
3. To achieve perfect proportions, it isn't enough to lose weight and develop and tone muscles; we must get hold of some of the fat and actually *redistribute* it to other, desirable areas.

What we didn't suspect at that point was a side effect of tremendous importance (one that you'll readily appreciate if you ever managed to lose weight only to gain it back as soon as you relaxed your vigilance): that by deliberately building up the fat deposits in certain desirable areas, such as the breasts, we would automatically guard against regaining weight we had managed to lose from hips, thighs, and other problem areas! Here is how it works.

How Balanced Physical Proportions Help You to Stay Slim and Shapely . . . Keep You from Regaining Flab You Had Lost

Under ordinary conditions, when healthy laboratory rats are allowed to feed as much as they want of a normally nutritious diet, they neither lose nor gain weight, proving the theory that in a normal individual the body itself regulates food intake to meet its needs. The question naturally arises, what part of the body is the key to this regulating system?

Here's an interesting phenomenon: In scientific experiments, pairs of healthy laboratory rats were surgically joined so that their brains received joint messages. When one of a pair was deliberately made voracious and obese through surgical lesions, the normal partner reduced its food intake or stopped eating altogether and continued to remain thin. Such feedback control regulating food intake seems to indicate that *signals from the fat depot affect the appetite-regulating centers.* In its reference to the work of Dr. David Levitsky, whose research is sponsored by the Weight Watchers Foundation, Consumer Guide's "Rating The Diets" states: "His research indicates that the *body's fat depots* send out messages to the hypothalamus, which *totals up* body fat and increases or decreases appetite accordingly."* (Italics are mine.)

Most of us thirty-seven women engaged in our experiments had at some time in our lives lost weight only to regain it as soon as we let up on our strict dieting, yet we successfully retained our new slim figures as soon as we were able to *balance* our total body fat according to our selected pattern. In other words, in the past, when we had lost weight all over, we were nicely slim in some parts but actually *underweight,* for our body requirements, in others. This was both unattractive to look at and unsatisfactory for the body's needs, and in fact our bodies quickly set to

*"Regulation of Adiposity and the Control of Food Intake," presented by Doctor David Levitsky at the First Annual Meeting of the American Society of Clinical Nutrition and the American Institute of Nutrition at Cornell University, August 14-17, 1973.

work restoring the former conditions. But when having first shed all excess weight and then further slimmed the parts that needed slimming and balanced the fat-loss by building up the rest of our shape, we looked terrific, our bodies were satisfied, and we remained slim and deliriously happy!

I suspect that this truth has crossed the minds of countless other figure experts, but aside from plastic surgery, when it is done with silicone and will not fool the body, as far as we know no one before us had the drive and the dedication to discover a method that would shape the female fat-cushions at will. It took thirty-seven vitally involved women three years of relentless idea-gathering, scientific research, and rigorous testing to perfect our method.

Something Old . . . Something New—but Nothing Blue!

These days scientists, nutritionists, and medical men are investigating more and more the remedies of the past, often finding scientific truth in tribal medicines or old wives' tales. Aside from searching the pages of the latest scientific publications, we also plundered annals of folklore, the memories of our elders, and the history books. When an idea seemed to hold promise, we divided into groups and gave the idea prolonged testing, with control groups to avoid errors. Only if the idea proved significantly effective did we accept it for scientific investigation, seeking to find out *why* it worked. With this system, only those methods that (a) worked, (b) were scientifically plausible, and (c) medically safe were incorporated into our program. They also had to be simple and pleasant, and where food was concerned, it had to be tasty and filling. After all, we were a basically lazy, food-loving lot!

Without going into the more unusual and scientifically complex items at this stage, let me give you an example.

The Case of the Identical Twins

In a scientific study on heredity versus environment, young Di happened to read about a pair of identical twins, orphan girls who had been brought up by families of different ethnic backgrounds. Among other "acquired tastes," one of the twins had developed a liking for strongly spiced, "hot" foods, while her sister preferred the bland cuisine on which her adopted family had raised her. In most other aspects they demonstrated remarkable resemblances, including the fact that they were both obese, and both were desperately trying to reduce. They were placed on identical diets.

What had caught Di's attention was this: Twin No. One complained that even though she stuck to the diet as faithfully as did her sister, and also did the same amount of exercises, she failed to lose weight as rapidly as Twin No. Two. She felt this was particularly unfair, since she happened to dislike the diet intensely, while her sister loved it.

This seemed strange to Di, for it is only logical that a meal you enjoy is better digested than a meal you dislike, and therefore, since more of the nutrients are utilized, should be more fattening. We all thought this was worth investigating.

We selected two groups of four women each, all with efficient digestions, and put both groups on identical 1,000-calorie diets planned around a few strong spices that one group loved, the other hated. In every other aspect, the two groups and their activities were as closely matched as was possible.

After eight weeks, the happy spice-lovers reported a combined weight-loss of 31 pounds, while the other group lost only a collective 19! Over the three-year period the experiment was repeated a number of times with different people and with different basic diets, and each time the result was the same: The group that loved the diet, no matter what it consisted of, succeeded in losing more weight than the group that did not enjoy it. (Providing, of course, that they consumed identical amounts.)

Under less controlled circumstances, the explanation would be simple: If you're deprived of eating satisfaction, you tend to nibble, continually seeking gustatory gratification and usually finding it in forbidden cookies and the like. But both in the case of the twins and our own experiments, we were satisfied that the 1,000-calorie per day diet was adhered to by all concerned. What, then, was the scientific explanation for this phenomenon?

It seems that eating meals you dislike not only inhibits the flow of digestive juices, but also causes *stress*. To manufacture the hormones produced during stress, the body uses up vitamins and minerals, making them unavailable to help convert body fat to energy. Hence, even though some reducing diets advocate dull foods in the hope that lack of enjoyment will result in lowered food intake, you'll actually *lose more fat eating meals you enjoy*—a conclusion we gladly incorporated into our method, as you will see in our chapter on diet and in the recipes!

There's an important lesson to be learned from this experiment, one that explains the seeming paradoxes of the Reshape Method, namely that enjoyable circumstances, great meals, pleasant exercise, and good relaxation will help you both to *trim off* fat and to *shape on* fat, depending on which aim you're working on. Simply put, bright spirits lead to success, misery leads to failure. That's why the Reshape Method tries to provide the most pleasant and rewarding conditions and materials to carry you happily toward your goals!

What Will Your Figure Be Like a Few Weeks From Today?

It took centuries of genetic coincidences, nine months of fetal development, and years of living to shape your body the way it is. Of course, the Reshape Program will not make you actually taller or shorter, nor will it give you longer legs or really narrow hips if your bones are short or wide—in short, it will not in any way change your bone structure. But you'll be amazed at how much it *can* do to actually change your figure type, give you smooth, slim lines, terrific posture, shapely limbs, and soft, feminine curves. In just a few weeks, you may undo almost all of those past influences and have the fabulous figure you always dreamed about and develop the slim, sexy lines you envied in others.

4

How the Reshape Program Works—The Science Behind the Magic

Everything you actually have to *do* to gain your fabulous new figure is set out for you in the easy, step-by-step summaries at the end of each section. Once you understand the principles behind the Reshape Program, you'll need only to glance at the numbered sequence to be able to follow through to your fabulous goals. But for the moment, let's look into the science behind the magic and find out how and why the Reshape Method really works.

Our chief aim is to manipulate *fat,* so we must first of all understand something of its nature and its place in the organism as a whole.

Fat as Storage of Energy and as Insulation

Deposited fat consists essentially of cells, which are just droplets of fat surrounded by a thin membranous shell of protoplasm. A man weighing 150 pounds has about 20 pounds of fat. A woman has quite a lot more.

Is there a need for this much adipose tissue (as fat is scientifically known)? Probably not. The role of fat is primarily that of storage of energy and of insulation, both abundantly important under primitive conditions, but not nearly so vital, at least in such quantities, in modern situations.

The advantage of fat as storage of energy is obvious: Fat contains no water, therefore it takes up little space, while it yields over twice as much energy as sugar. (One gram of fat yields nine calories, one gram of either protein or carbohydrate yields only four.) Also, for the most part fat stays liquid at body temperature. It is therefore quite clear that primitive man, often in need of large infusions of energy while hunting his prey over difficult terrain, had reason to be thankful for those fatty deposits that, without hindering his movements, provided him when times were hard with up to forty days of metabolic energy. Similarly, early man—the most naked of mammals—needed subcutaneous fat to insulate him from heat and from the cold.

Today, food is only as far as the pizza parlor or the refrigerator. Clothes protect us from the elements. We know, in fact, that excess weight is not only unattractive, but actually dangerous to our health. All the same, we need some reserve energy stored in our fat depots to provide us with our continuous energy needs between meals, and we need some padding to cushion our bones and our organs from injuries, to protect us from extremes in temperature, and in the case of women, to give us pleasing feminine contours. Moreover, scientists believe that energy storage and insulation are not the only roles fat plays in the life of the organism.

The Function of Fat as a Metabolic Organ

Recent scientific studies indicate that far from being merely a static store of energy and insulation, fat is in fact an organ of high metabolic activity, with a considerable oxygen uptake and a rapid rate of turnover. Half the adipose tissue of normal rats is metabolized and reconstituted in five to nine days. A middle-aged woman weighing 130 pounds would be forming and destroying about 3 pounds of fat every twenty-four hours.

Based on this evidence, scientists believe that adipose tissue must be taking part in the day-to-day energy exchanges of the organism as a whole. Moreover, as we have seen in the case of the surgically joined rats, recent studies indicate that adipose tissue may itself be responsible for the messages to the brain controlling appetite, dictated either by total adipose volume, or by fat-cell size.

The Fat-for-Energy Exchange

The food we eat provides us not only with the building blocks the body needs to build new body structures, but also with the energy to do the building. When more food is taken in than needed, the excess is turned into glycogen, a small emergency-supply in the liver and muscles; the rest is stored as fat. When less is taken than needed, the additional energy requirements are withdrawn from the fat depots. (The exception is energy for the brain and nervous system, which cannot utilize fat for energy and must be supplied at such times from the emergency glycogen reserves.)

A common misconception relating to the fat-for-energy system is that this energy input/output is a very simple equation, something similar to money deposited and then withdrawn from the bank. The fact is that if our banks behaved the way our bodies do, our fortunes would not be in very safe hands. For the body doesn't care about honorable finances—what it cares about most is its own economy, the most efficient and cheapest (in terms of energy expenditure) way it can carry out its functions. It shrewdly watches its energy expenditure and if the need arises, adjusts its metabolism to fit the circumstances. (For instance, some authorities calculate that it takes a 3,500-calorie deficit to lose one pound, but only 2,500 surplus calories to gain one! Talk about injustice!) Consequently, if you want to lose weight fast, it is not enough to know how many calories you have to cut and how much you should exercise—the real trick is getting your body to give up the most fat in the shortest time with the least effort. When it comes to the fat that matters—the *bulk* fat—that's not an easy thing to do.

What is Bulk Fat?

Most dietary fat is carried first in the lymphatic circulation and from there into the bloodstream, where substances in the blood break it down. Smaller fat particles are literally absorbed into the fat cells and into the liver. Others are processed so that they can be used by the cells of the body for energy. What is not used is then returned to the bloodstream to be carried to the fat cells for storage. The same happens to fat converted from excess carbohydrates and even from excess protein.

Since the bloodstream serves as its transportation system, it's not surprising that fat cells in the region of high blood flow are the first to take up and to release fat content, while the bulk of adipose tissue remains more constant. In fact, scientists suggest that human adipose tissue is made up of two distinct stores: one, the smaller pool, utilized in our day-to-day metabolism, while the other, the bulk pool, is called upon only in times of extreme need, such as starvation. Our own findings were that under ordinary weight-control regimes we tended to lose—gain—lose—gain in the same regions, without making much of a dent where it really mattered: in our main bulk fat. It was when we learned to mobilize the fat from our main, bulk fat stores that we began to see amazing results.

How Bulk Fat Gets to be Deposited, and Where—and Why?

Like any solid or semisolid substance carried in a liquid medium, fat tends to settle (1) where circulation takes it, (2) where there's room to settle, and (3) where it can flourish undisturbed.

CIRCULATION

The heart pumps fresh oxygenated blood through the arteries. Arteries branch into arterioles, which in turn branch into the capillaries. The capillary walls are only one cell thin, thus allowing nutrients and oxygen to pass through, and waste materials to seep back into the bloodstream. While arterial blood is pumped at high pressure, the return, or venous, blood pressure through the venules and then through the veins back to the heart is pretty low. Under these conditions it isn't difficult to appreciate that over long periods of time, through hindering the blood flow, *the effects of gravity cause fat to accumulate over the lower part of the body.*

The same is true of any other circumstance hindering return blood flow, such as constriction of blood vessels due to tight pantyhose or to the steady pressure of a chair seat against a secretary's fanny. (Naturally, those with "android" type constitutions will not be so affected, since they have no appreciable quantities of fat cells in the lower body to begin with. In men, the lowest that gravity will pull the fat is generally to the paunch.)

WHERE THERE IS ROOM TO SETTLE

Contrary to the above—and this may seem like something of a paradox—a tight garment may sometimes *hinder* the deposition of fat, by not allowing enough room for it to settle. Pressure from without or from within, such as of tight belts, bandages, *tight wedding rings,* or even of pregnancy or tumor, "all reduce locally the accumulation of subcutaneous fat, as if displacing it toward the periphery of the pressure area."*

Another kind of internal pressure depriving fat of room to settle is muscle—the space between bulging biceps and taut skin just isn't enough for large deposits of fat to form.

*Albert E. Renold and George F. Cahill, Jr., eds., Section 5 "Adipose Tissue" in *Handbook of Physiology* (Washington, D.C.: American Physiological Society, 1965).

WHERE FAT CAN FLOURISH UNDISTURBED

For the deposited fat to become the unyielding mass of *bulk* fat, it must be undisturbed; the longer it remains so, the more entrenched it will become.

The lack of vigorous return blood flow is one reason why fat remains undisturbed. Another is lack of nerve stimulus. For instance, injury to a nerve is usually followed by accumulation of fat in the denervated area. Over the abdomen, lack of tone of the abdominal muscles is a frequent cause of fat.

Hormonal influences play their part as well, and so does enzyme activity. The body manufactures enzymes to bring about countless metabolic actions. Economical as always, the body will not produce in large numbers those enzymes for which there is no frequent call. If your energy needs are customarily met from newly synthetized materials from food, and hardly ever from *stored* fat, then the enzymes necessary for processing stored fat into energy will be in short supply. The more you burn fat, the more fat you'll burn. In the course of our lengthy and often repeated experiments, as time went by many of us found that we could produce much greater fat-loss in much less time than we had been able to at the beginning of our project, even when the technique and other conditions were the same.

Finally, temperature may also play a part in solid fat formation. Although most human fat is liquid at body temperature, some fat components are less so, and these may be responsible for helping fat to solidify in certain areas close to the surface of the skin, especially if exposed to cold. Also, by prompting the body to provide extra insulation, cold could attract the accumulation of fat to frequently exposed areas.

One important point to remember is that newly laid down deposits of fat need not necessarily originate from newly synthetized fat from food, but may come from fat circulating in the blood as a result of vigorous exercise or even *as a result of dieting!*

When energy needs cannot be met from newly synthetized food sources and are instead satisfied by breaking down stored fat, the resulting circulating fat, if not all burned up, may simply find its way to a new storage site and settle there. This may explain why it sometimes happens that on a weight-loss program you lose fat from your chest and *actually gain some on your buttocks!*

5

The Tools of the Reshape Program

Marvelous and mysterious as the body is, it quite readily responds to the simplest mechanical and chemical influences. If you lower your head, blood will flow to your brain. If you apply cold to your skin, surface blood vessels will contract. If you eat a lot of salt, your tissues will retain fluid, just like your salt shaker. In the Reshape Program we naturally make use of diet and exercise, but in conjunction with such influences as gravity, compression, pressure, stimulation, heat, cold, friction, circulation, and more. But none of these would be of much use without a fair understanding of the mechanics and chemistry of digestion (taking into account its various stages and their durations), and absorption.

Digestion

The process of digestion starts in the mouth. Food ground into smaller particles by the teeth is lubricated by the saliva, while the enzyme amylase in the saliva begins to chemically break down starch. The food bolus is then passed along the esophagus toward the stomach. Automatic wavelike contractions, called peristalsis, help propel the food toward the stomach even if you are in the horizontal position. In the presence of hydrochloric acid in the stomach the enzyme pepsin begins to break down protein into smaller units. As the enzyme amylase cannot act in the presence of a strong acid such as hydrochloric acid, the digestion of starch is temporarily suspended until the food, now churned to a semiliquid mass called chyme, is passed on into the small intestine. Here alkaline juices neutralize the acid, and carbohydrate digestion can proceed. In the small intestine the chyme is mixed with bile from the liver, and with the juices from the pancreas and those formed within the intestine. Enzymes in the digestive juices break proteins down into their component amino acids, carbohydrates into simple sugars, and fats into glycerol and free fatty acids. Now the amino acids from the proteins and the simple sugars from the carbohydrates are absorbed through the walls of the small intestine into the small surrounding veins to be passed on into the bloodstream. Most of the fat is picked up by the second circulatory system, the lymphatics, to be also emptied eventually into the bloodstream, while indigestible residues such as cellulose are passed on to the large intestine to be eliminated eventually. The entire process from ingestion to elimination may last forty-eight hours or longer. Of this time, the food spends four to five hours in the stomach from where very little absorption takes place, and a further two to ten hours in the small intestine, which is about twenty-two feet long, and from where most of the nutrients are absorbed into the bloodstream. The longest sojourn, mostly of waste products, is in the large intestines, awaiting elimination and absorbing water.

The rate of digestion and absorption depends mainly on just what is being digested. Obviously, solid foods take longer than liquid or semiliquid, as they have to be homogenized in the stomach before they can be passed on to the small intestine. Proteins, too, must spend time in the stomach, as their chemical breakdown begins there. On the other hand, carbohydrates, whose breakdown had started in the mouth, are passed directly into the small intestine for final breakdown. Carbohydrate digestion is fastest, protein digestion takes longer, fat digestion takes longest. Coldness slows down the process, warmth speeds it up. Therefore, a cold, fatty solid takes the longest time

to digest, while a warm, sweet liquid passes almost directly into the bloodstream.

The food now circulating in the bloodstream will provide the cells with the building blocks they need to build new body structures and also with the energy they need to do the building. The amino acids from the proteins are the main building blocks; carbohydrates in the form of the simple sugar glucose provide the energy. Glucose not immediately used is partly stored in the liver and muscles as glycogen to be released as needed in case of emergency, while the rest is converted and stored as fat. Within about thirteen hours of the last replacement of glucose, all available supplies (with the exception of the glycogen) have been used up.

It is at this point that if no new supplies of glucose are introduced the body turns to its fat stores for needed energy.

The Role of Hormones in Controlling Blood Sugar

The body keeps the amount of glucose in the blood within quite narrow limits by raising or lowering glucose levels as needed. To raise the level, it can take glucose from carbohydrates in the diet, or from liver glycogen, or it can convert glycerol from fat into glucose. The glycerol of 100 grams of fat provides 12 grams of glucose. While fat's other constituents, the fatty acids, cannot be converted to glucose, they can help to maintain blood glucose levels by providing energy, thereby sparing available blood glucose.

To lower blood glucose levels if they're excessive, the body can use several means:

1. Convert glucose to glycogen. Only a limited amount of glycogen can be stored in the liver and muscles for future use.
2. Step up expenditure of energy.
3. *Convert glucose to fat.*

(When blood glucose levels are much too high to process in these manners, the body simply spills some of the blood glucose over into the kidneys from where it is excreted in the urine.)

Several hormones help increase the blood sugar level, while it is the job of the hormone *insulin* to help decrease it.

Whenever you eat something that causes the blood sugar level to rise, there'll be a sharp outpouring of insulin to help lower it again. If it falls too much, insulin production will lessen and other hormones will pour out to raise the level of glucose in the blood. In this manner, a healthy person's blood sugar will remain at desirable levels most of the time.

One way insulin helps to lower the blood glucose level is by actively promoting the conversion of glucose into fatty acids. Scientists have actually proved that high insulin levels promote the deposition of fat, while low levels of insulin promote the mobilization of fat. In fact, laboratory experiments have shown that liver treated with insulin will speed up fatty acid formation to a great extent, while diabetic rat liver slices, which have no insulin action, cannot form fatty acids at all.

From the above it will readily be seen that for successful weight control, it isn't only *what* we do but *when* we do it that matters. Even on a low-food-intake/high-energy-output regime

MOST FAT WILL BE BURNED	LEAST FAT WILL BE BURNED
1. when low blood sugar forces body to burn stored energy	1. when raised blood sugar from dietary source satisfies energy needs
2. when low insulin level *promotes* mobilization of fat from stores.	2. when raised insulin level *prohibits* mobilization of fat from stores.

The jogger who jogs late in the day or the tennis player who plays two grueling sets two to three hours after breakfast, will achieve twice the effect with half the effort once she learns the few simple truths of the Woman's Total Reshape Program.

Distribution of Meals

Scientists have found evidence that the daily distribution of meals may also have something to do with the formation of adipose tissue. Rats fed one large meal a day seem to store more fat than rats allowed to feed the same quantity of food throughout the day. This finding, however, seems to apply principally to meals consisting of large amounts of carbohydrate. It seems that the enzymes that help to store fat, and that under normal conditions adapt themselves to varying sized meals, under conditions of starvation tend to *atrophy* (waste away), while, on the other hand, repeated large meals of carbohydrates result in *hypertrophy* of these enzymes, causing them to be exceptionally active. We will discuss the question of the traditional meal plan versus the newer six-or-more-small-meals concept in a later chapter.

Diet—Should You Worry about Your "Ideal Weight"?

Judy and Helen are both five feet six inches tall. At the beginning of our experiments, Judy weighed 145 pounds, Helen weighed only 130. Both were overweight, Judy more so than Helen, yet Judy's figure was infinitely nicer than Helen's. Why? Simply because Judy was more attractively proportioned.

In the Woman's Reshape Program we make use of "ideal" weights only as a rough guide and as an important tool in calculating calorie requirements.

For your ideal weight allow 100 pounds for 5 feet of your height, plus three more pounds for every additional inch, minus 1 pound for every two years you're under twenty-five years old.

If the above is lower than most charts you've consulted in the past, remember, we're not just aiming for a reasonably attractive figure, we're absolutely determined to shape your figure to as near film-star proportions as your bone structure permits. While low body weight alone doesn't automatically give you a film-star figure, it gets you a fair distance of the way.

How About "Type of Build"?

I know that on most charts you have a choice of three "ideal weights": for slight frame, for medium frame, and for large frame. Well, unless you're extremely small- or large-boned, forget it. Most of us fall into the medium build category—if you're the least bit unsure, then so do you. A reasonable guide to type of frame is your wrist measurement: substantially under 6 inches (measured right on the wrist bone) means you are small-boned. Substantially over 6½ inches, you're probably large-framed. In these cases you may deduct or add to your ideal weight up to about six or seven pounds. Let's say you're a girl of nineteen standing five feet six in your bare feet, with a wrist measurement of 6½ inches; your ideal weight is

First 5 feet of height	100 pounds
3 pounds per each extra inch	+18
Minus 1 pound per each two years you're under twenty-five	− 3
	Ideal weight 115 pounds

Since your wrist measures just 6½ inches, you're not sufficiently heavy-framed to earn you any extra allowance.

On the other hand, if you're thirty-five years old, 5 feet tall, and your wrist measures 5½ inches, then your ideal weight is one hundred pounds, less about *three* pounds for being extra small-boned. On the other hand, should you be exceptionally large-boned (wrist substantially above 6½ inches), then you may add *five or six* pounds to your chart weight, because the difference in bone-weight is greater in your case than in the case of the small-framed person.

Firm Tissue is Heavier Than "Flab"

Remember two important points: (1) Firm, taut tissue weighs more than flab, so the chart allowances here provide for an even slimmer, trimmer shape than the figures would indicate, and (2) your ideal weight is merely a guide to find the proper tool you're going to use for your figure-shaping program. The aim is to make you slim, svelte, taut, and terrific, not to win a featherweight championship! When you've reached your ideal *measurements,* when your mirror tells you that you're stupendous, and admiring glances confirm it, *that* will be your "ideal weight," even if it's five or six pounds over—or under—what the chart indicates.

For the moment, though, let's concentrate on the ideal weight result. Whether you weigh more than you should, in which case first of all you must lose weight fast, or your weight is right or even *under* the ideal but your shape is wrong, your ideal weight result will give us an important "tool" to work with: your daily calorie need.

Calories—You Probably Know All About Them

If you're like nine out of ten American women, you've read hundreds of magazine articles and books on the role of calories in weight reduction. You know that a calorie is a unit used by scientists to measure the energy yielded by the various foods when they're burned (metabolized) in the body. If you consume more calories than your system burns, you'll store the excess as fat. If you consume less, you'll shed the difference. You also know that to lose one pound of fat, you must consume about 3,500 calories less than your body's energy needs. In other words, to lose one pound a week, you must consume daily 500 calories less than your normal calorie requirement. It seems a simple enough mathematical exercise; why is it then that millions of words are written about the subject month after month, and still millions of people are walking about, dragging their unwanted fat?

Part of the reason is that most reducing diets are so unsatisfying, people just don't stay on them. Who can spend a life-time on one-ounce portions of this or that anemic-looking stuff and a bunch of celery sticks? As for the gelatin desserts, the fake mousses, and other lo-cal meal extenders, our systems must be crying out against synthetic products that try to fool our palates but cannot fool our bodies! With the Reshape Diet, I can promise you this: Your eyes, your nose, and your palate will be thrilled and your stomach satisfied. Your plate brimming with rich-tasting food, you can sit at the table with your partners without that "deprived" feeling and can rise from it as fulfilled and as well—or better—nourished as they are. In fact, they'll be asking to eat the same.

Another reason why you'll find it easy to stay with the Reshape Program is the fact that it is a *total* concept, not just a diet or exercise routine to lose weight. You'll be so involved, your mind will be so eager and occupied that it'll have less time or inclination to dwell on mere food.

The fact is that the body's arithmetic is not the same as that of an adding machine. A computer would be a closer analogy, for innumerable factors influence the outcome of each and every biological operation. That juicy steak 300 calories over and above your day's calorie requirement could end up as an extra layer of fat on your tummy, or it could go to build some vital tissue, or else it could actually help your body to burn unwanted fat. Conversely, that 500-calorie deficit you count on slimming your waistline could do just that, or it could tear down some shapely muscle, or it could even cause more fat than you burn to be released into the bloodstream, resulting in damage to arteries or to liver, or in a freshly deposited layer of fat where you least want it! The Reshape Program feeds infinitely more input material into the "computer" than just food, which is also why its results are so rewarding.

All the same, even though calories alone are far from being the last word in figure control, like "ideal weight," your "ideal calorie requirements" are also an important guideline, and a tool with which you'll be working.

YOUR DAILY CALORIE NEEDS

		12
YOUR		(If you're under fifty)
"IDEAL	X	11
WEIGHT"		(If you're over fifty)
	+	5% if very active
		10% if extremely active

Your Daily Calorie Needs

To get your daily calorie need, multiply your "ideal weight" by 12 if you're under fifty, by 11 if you're over. Again we're being stingier than most diet guides, but we want to become terrific, not just less fat. If you're very vigorously active—run two miles a day plus play an hour of squash or similar sport—then you may add 5 to 10 percent, depending on how very vigorously active you are. Example: Your "ideal weight" is 115 pounds, you're thirty-two years old, and you work in an office; you do yoga once a week and play golf on the weekends. Your calorie requirement: $115 \times 12 = 1,380$ calories.

To consume 500 calories less than the 1,380 you need to maintain your weight once you've reached it, your total intake for the time being must be no more than 900 calories. In terms of the traditional three meals a day, that's pretty skimpy indeed.

Most 900-Calorie Diets Are for the Birds

"Use small plates so the meal will *seem* bigger . . . eat slowly, so it'll last longer . . ." are the tips most diet guides give to ease the torture. Of course, these measures won't do any harm, but they're not going to make a food-loving, hollow-stomached dieter either full or happy. Nor are they going to keep her on the diet very long. In efforts to overcome the problem, various lopsided diets have been advocated, but it is best to steer clear of them because they're unpleasant and may well be dangerous.

You Must Have a Well-Balanced Diet

First of all, you must realize that regardless of whether they come from proteins, carbohydrates, or fats, excess calories will turn into excess poundage—so there's no way that you can gorge yourself on any kind of food with impunity if it means your total calorie intake will be higher than your needs. It may be true that protein digestion itself burns slightly more energy than carbohydrate digestion, for instance, but the difference is negligible (at most about an additional one and a half ounces per week), while excessively high protein diets may be damaging to the kidneys.

Remember also, dieting and exercise result in increased fatty acids in the blood—a condition many doctors consider undesirable. That is the more reason why we must eat the right foods: They will provide us with the vitamins and minerals that are so indispensable for burning fatty acids and thereby disposing of them.

There are many nutrients the body cannot store. These must be supplied day by day in adequate amounts. The less you eat, the less chance there is for all these nutrients to be supplied in the quantities they're needed. That's why even a 900-calorie diet may be deficient, and why many doctors recommend that you take vitamin and mineral supplements while you're dieting. If your doctor is of the opinion that while you're on the Aussie Reshape diet you should have extra vitamins and minerals, then by all means take them. Most of us, however, did not take any supplements; here's why.

Nutritionists are constantly discovering new constituents in our foods that are essential to our well-being and hitherto unsuspected roles for others, so that there is no definite answer to the question, what is needed and what is not? Furthermore, in the presence of some nutrients, the need for others increases. Some interact unfavorably with others—and so on. All this points to the fact that getting your vitamins and minerals from nature's own foods makes sense: In a balanced diet, these nutrients are supplied in sufficient quantities and in the correct proportions and combinations, ensuring good health, more efficient digestion, and more effortless and successful fat-burning. It also stands to reason that the more nutrients your food contains, the less food you need to eat. Hence, less calories are needed.

Fortunately, in the long run a balanced diet seems to be the only *possible* diet. Lopsided diets, apart from promoting ill health, often fail because our bodies refuse them. Our system is equipped with automatic controls: We *need* balanced nutrition, therefore most often we crave it. No matter how much you may love steak, if all you're allowed is meat, you'll soon be longing for a potato, or a bowl of crisp greens, or a juicy apple. No matter how sweet your tooth, a steady diet of cakes and candy would soon make you clamor for a piece of roast or a hunk of cheese. So the only sensible way, in fact the only possible way to diet is by consuming the necessary proteins, fats, and carbohydrates with vitamins and minerals plentifully supplied. That's why in the Reshape Diet we insisted not only on great taste and great fill-power, but also on superior all-round nutrition.

Some Foods Are Less Fattening than Others—But Who Wants to Nibble on a Plateful of Lettuce?

Weight for weight, fat has two and one-fourth times as many calories as either proteins or carbohydrates. Vitamins and minerals have none. But we don't eat proteins, fats, carbohydrates, vitamins, and minerals; we eat *foods* that contain often all of these nutrients in varying proportions—plus *water*. It is the water content of foods that determines how fattening they are, for the simple reason that water has no calories. Fats, which contain little or no water, are the most fattening of foods and nonstarchy vegetables such as cucumber or lettuce are the least fattening, since they may contain as much as 95 percent water, plus undigestible fiber. Next on the list are fruits and starchy vegetables, then lean meats, then fatty meats, then fats such as butter or margarine (which also have some 15 to 20 percent water). It isn't hard to guess then which would fill up a large empty plate more: one third of one small hamburger or thirty-three stalks of asparagus (both approximately 100 calories). The trouble is that a limp broccoli or a dry lettuce leaf is cold comfort indeed. Even those who like vegetables consider them as merely side dishes, and as for salads, without liberal amounts of oily dressings, they've become the very symbols of deprived dieting. Yet it is clear that this is where the answer lies: If we want to have our plates richly piled and our stomachs well satisfied, we must fill them with the foods that provide the largest amounts of bulk at the lowest caloric values. The question we asked ourselves over and over: How can we make vegetables look, smell, and taste so delicious that we'll want to eat huge amounts of them and never tire.

In German It's Gemüse, in Hungarian, It's Fözelék

The Chinese fry their vegetables; the French, though they hold them in great esteem, still consider them a side dish. The Italians mostly mix them with fattening pasta. But several of our group who were of middle-European ancestry remembered the large plates of German *Gemüse* or Hungarian *fözelék* they had often eaten in their grandparents' homes. These man-sized dishes, which were accompanied by small portions of meat, poultry, or even by just a couple of fried or poached eggs, were prepared in special, rich-tasting and filling ways and served as main dishes at almost every meal. So out came Grandmother's cookbooks, and dozens of truly delicious and wonderfully satisfying dishes have been on our menu ever since. The beauty of these dishes is that when the big bulk of your diet is so low in calories, you can afford the extras that add the yummy touches. The Hungarians especially are fond of rich food, and many of these recipes call for such luxuries as sour cream. Since a whole pound of most vegetables contributes only about 100 calories (often even less), we have been able to include even such rich fare as sour cream in our diet.

Served following a clear broth, these huge platefuls of vegetable dishes, with a portion of fish or poultry, and a fruit dessert, add up to an eye-filling, plate-filling, stomach-filling meal at about 400 calories. What is more, some vegetables—cabbage in particular—seem to possess a fat-mobilizing property science may not be able to explain but which we have found to be very real. Given two diets with identical calorie content but differing ingredients, the one that is built mainly around vegetables will take weight off at a much faster rate than the other. Raw vegetables work particularly well, perhaps because of their high vitamin, mineral, and enzyme content. As in our recipes, however, the cooking water is included in the rich sauce, none of these valuable nutrients get spilled down the drain.

We have also found a way to make wonderfully rich-tasting cream soups at very low calories. These soups make an ideal lunch meal on their own.

What we have tried to do is avoid that hungry, miserable feeling of *deprivation* most dieters seem to suffer. Our meals are big, satisfying, and they shun substitutions, artificial ingredients, fake foods, and mock delicacies that set the dieter apart from her peers. I know you'll enjoy them as much as we did!

Frequent Small Meals vs. Traditional Meal Plan

Lately it has been advocated that as many as six small meals—barely more than snacks—should take the place of the traditional three meals (with lunch and dinner the main meals) each day. Also, it has been suggested that breakfast should be the most substantial of the meals, with each subsequent meal lighter than the one before.

Our findings suggest otherwise.

You will remember I have already mentioned that scientific evidence confirms that repeated very large carbohydrate loads cause hypertrophy of the fat-converting enzymes—in other words, after large carbohydrate meals, these enzymes work overtime stacking fat into the fat cells. This may very well be the case when large quantities of spaghetti or pie are consumed, but while our low-starch vegetables are classified as carbohydrate foods, their actual carbohydrate content is very small. One pound of asparagus contains not much more than 20 grams of carbohydrate, one pound of spinach contains even less. In actual fact, while a single average hamburger (a "protein" food) may contain as many as 32 grams of carbohydrate, a huge plateful of one of our delicious vegetable dishes contains no more than 20!

We have found that frequent eating makes dieting sheer torture. With such tiny "meals" you never feel really satisfied, and your mind is constantly on food. No sooner have you swallowed (often in one bite) one so-called meal, than you're already watching the clock in anticipation of the next. Also, we have found that frequent eating leads to frequent unplanned nibbling, which taken all together can add up to many times the permitted calories. With the Reshape Program, when we have finished one large, satisfying meal, we brush our teeth or rinse our mouth and put all thought of food from our minds until the next meal.

As for breakfast to be the most substantial meal, here too we disagree, our opinions based on both scientific fact and on our own findings.

To digest a large meal, the system must divert a large portion of its blood flow to the stomach and the intestines. Other organs, notably the brain, are then deprived of their full quotas, which is why we feel drowsy after a large meal. Mornings, which are generally busy periods whether at work or at home or out shopping, are hardly suited to peaceful, undisturbed digestion. It's not for nothing that in most cultures the main meal of the day is eaten in the evening, or, as in some parts of Europe, at midday followed by a two-hour siesta!

Psychologically, too, the traditional sequence of small break-fast, light lunch, and substantial evening meal seems to be the ideal one. Many people don't even feel hungry in the morning, certainly not hungry enough for the biggest meal of the day! By lunchtime, we're a little more relaxed and we enjoy our lunch. But best of all we enjoy our meals in the evening, when most of us are at home with hours to while away. Just think of it: If you ate your main meal in the morning, in a hurry, and without even feeling hungry, and your next most substantial meal at still-busy lunchtime, then you'd have to face the rest of the day and the evening with a feeling that—at least from the standpoint of food—you have nothing more to look forward to! And you would have several hungry hours to spend in the close proxim-ity of the kitchen, or even *in* it, handling food, tasting it for flavor, serving it to your family! In our opinion a modest breakfast (if any), a filling but light lunch, and a whopping big, rich, satisfying dinner make for happy dieters!

For the success of the Reshape Program, however, it doesn't really matter which of your meals is the main meal. If you personally prefer a big breakfast and are content with a lesser lunch and a still less substantial dinner, that's just fine. As long as you keep to the permitted calories, and as long as you *eat or drink absolutely nothing until at least a half hour after your morning exercises!* Why? You'll find out in a minute.

Exercise

In the Reshape Program we've tried to make this terrific body-shaping process as painless as humanly possible, and to most of us thirty-seven lazy ladies, any exercise seemed verging on sheer physical torture. Have we been able to eliminate it from our program? Frankly, no. But we've found ways to wring every last drop of benefit from the relatively few and unexhausting routines we have included, and we have managed to make them quite comfortable and pleasant.

Why Exercise?

There's no question about it, exercise is healthy, and in our modern labor-saving society, for most people some form of routine daily exercise is a must. But as far as weight-reduction or figure-shaping is concerned, exercise generally has only limited application.

HELPS TO "BURN" FAT

It is true that by requiring additional energy and by increasing oxidation, exercise does help burn fat, but you'd have to do an awful lot of knee bends to make a real dent in your bulk fat stores! Ten minutes of running burns about a hundred calories, ten minutes of swimming only about 50 calories (though more if the water is *freezing!*). You would have to bicycle for about three hours every day to burn up the 500 calories that would add up to a mere one-pound loss per week. We of the Reshape Program believe in moderation, especially when we're dealing with something as uncongenial as exercise. If you enjoy strenuous and prolonged exercise, however, then just go right ahead and do it. It is good for you and it can only help. But it is certainly not a necessity.

EXERCISE TO "SPOT-REDUCE"

Many books and magazines recommend specific exercises to slim hips, thighs, waist, and so on. Others will just as emphatically inform you that "spot-reducing" is all bunkum. The truth, as is so often the case, may lie between the two. It is perfectly true that a muscle being exercised may call for fat to be released from the fat cells for energy. It is also perfectly true that the message the muscle sends out through hormonal and nervous signals goes to *all* the fat cells in the body and they *all* release a little of their fat content into the bloodstream to be transported to the particular muscle where additional energy is needed, resulting in a small uniform fat-loss all over the body and not just from the area where the muscle is being exercised. On the other hand, there's evidence that at least some of the additional energy may be supplied directly from the fat stored between the muscle fibers of the muscle being exercised. The effect is probably not substantial, but of course every little bit helps.

INCREASED MUSCLE MASS INCREASES BASAL METABOLISM

Another reason often put forward in favor of exercise for weight control is that muscle mass as such burns more energy than fat mass, and this is also true. This is one of the reasons why men can consume more calories than women without putting on extra weight. (Talk about equality of the sexes!) Their basic metabolic need is higher than ours because of their bigger muscle/fat ratio. But we do not wish to have the figure of male athletes, and so for us this argument, like the two previous ones, has only limited validity.

The Reshape Reasons for (moderate) Exercise

1. The combined effects of the Reshape Program will result in increased amounts of free fatty acids released from the fat stores into the bloodstream. If this fatty acid content of the blood is greater than the oxidative needs of the cells, then the excess may be stored in the various organs and cause such unhealthy consequences as fatty liver. Exercise will induce the extra oxidation necessary to avoid such a condition.

2. As we have said before, one of our principal tools in figure-shaping is *circulation*. Exercise helps to boost circulation and carry away the fat globules the other Reshape activities have freshly released from the bulk fat depots into the bloodstream.

3. When you exercise a particular muscle of your body, blood flow automatically is diverted to that muscle and away from other parts of your system whose needs are not as urgent. By relaxing the rest of your anatomy and concentrating your efforts on the selected part, you can direct greatly increased blood flow to wherever you want it—a great help in both the slimming and the building-up process.

4. As you remember, one of the means by which we can keep fat from settling in any area is by limiting the space where it can gather, either through external or internal means. We will use external methods at specific times and to a limited degree. But for permanence, nothing can make fat more uncomfortable than well-developed muscles crowding tightly against the skin.

5. Vigorous exercise after a twelve- or thirteen-hour fast, in other words, before you've had anything to eat or drink in the morning, is one of the Reshape Program's most important reducing tools.

Why Exercise on an Empty Digestive Tract?

As I mentioned before, the traditional reason why we should avoid exercise after we've eaten is increased activity necessitates increased blood flow. When you exercise, the energy needs of your muscles are paramount. Blood is directed to supply these needs at the expense of digestion, leaving digestion temporarily suspended. In general, you're advised not to undertake strenuous exercise for a half hour or an hour after you eat. In our opinion, since digestion is a much lengthier process, strenuous exercise would best be reserved for the pre-breakfast period when *no* digestion is taking place at all. But for the Reshape Method, there's a much more compelling reason, one to which we attribute a large measure of our success: *Before breakfast is a time of low insulin concentration.*

As you will remember, high concentrations of insulin in the blood not only promote the storage of fat in the fat cells, but in the presence of quantities of insulin the release and breakdown of fat actually can't take place. This means that even if through vigorous exercise the muscles' energy needs necessitate release of fat from the fat cells, the presence of large amounts of insulin in the blood will prevent this from happening. It stands to reason, consequently, that to gain real, substantial fat-reducing benefit from exercise, you must do it at a time when insulin production is at its lowest: in the morning, when blood glucose levels are at an ebb because you have had no nourishment since dinner the night before.

Even one glass of orange juice will boost the glucose level in your blood minutes after you drink it, resulting in an immediate outpouring of insulin into the bloodstream and in a blockage of the fat-release you're working so hard to achieve. In our experiments we have found that all other things being equal, up to 30 percent more weight was lost when exercises were performed in the morning before either food or drink was taken, than if the same kind and number of exercises were done at any other time of the day. Or, if you prefer it that way, the same weight-loss could be achieved with only 70 percent of the effort.

Naturally, as with any exercise program, you must consult your own doctor before you start. But you need not worry that exercising while your blood sugar is low will result in hypoglycemia. Remember, in a healthy person who has been eating an adequate diet, there are about 100 grams of glycogen stored in the liver—enough to supply glucose for the entire body's needs for two whole days in case of emergency. While in order to spare diminished glucose levels the muscles will be supplied with the energy they need from the fat depots, as is our aim, the brain and nervous system will get their glucose needs from the blood, and if that is not enough, then from the glycogen stored in the liver.

Types of Exercise

In the Woman's Reshape Program, we try to limit quantity, and concentrate on quality and type of exercise. Each kind we do serves a specific purpose.

EXERCISE TO BURN FAT FASTEST

The larger the muscle being exercised, the more energy it will require, and the more fat it will burn. The largest muscles are those that move the legs, and our experiments confirmed that exercises using those muscles (in hips, buttocks, and thighs) acted almost twice as fast burning up fat than did even hard exercises involving the upper body, such as push-ups. Our main choice is running and jumping.

EXERCISE TO INCREASE CIRCULATION

To keep those freshly released fat globules moving away from their favorite hiding places, we must make sure that blood is freely pumped into the remotest blood vessels, and flooding into the narrowest capillaries. For this we need fast, heart-thumping action and what is better suited to this purpose than running and jumping? So with one short daily running and jumping routine we achieve both of these important purposes.

EXERCISE FOR FLEXIBILITY

Muscles, ligaments, and tendons must be kept in flexible shape not only to keep blood freely circulating, but also to develop suppleness and grace. A few slow, lazy stretching routines are all that is needed.

EXERCISE FOR TONE

An important reason why fat may accumulate in a certain location, as you will remember, is lack of nerve stimulus in the particular area. One of the several ways in which the Reshape Method ensures good nerve stimulus and muscle tone is through the rhythmic movements of some quite simple calisthenics.

ENLARGING MUSCLES TO KEEP OUT FAT

This is how some body-building experts explain what makes a muscle grow: Severe strain on a muscle, such as in weight lifting, results first of all in a tearing down of muscle tissue. This may sound frightening, but there's no need to worry, for the nutrient-rich blood rushing to the site will immediately start to rebuild the muscle bigger and stronger than it was before.

In the Woman's Reshape Program, we also use isometric exercises and some mild weight-lifting to achieve the same results. Of course, we don't want to gain body-builder proportions, but we do want certain muscles to develop sufficiently so they will crowd into the spaces otherwise occupied by fat.

DIRECTING BLOOD FLOW

The same nutrient-rich blood that brings to the muscle the building blocks to create bigger and stronger tissue also carries fat globules or materials that may be converted to fat. For those of us who desire to enlarge our bust measurements, this is an important concept and unique to the Woman's Reshape Program. For this is one of the means by which we are able to direct the flow of the special Reshape nutrients toward their goal. Other bust development programs use rich nutrients in an effort to build up the breasts and they sometimes succeed, but they also succeed in adding extra inches to waist, hips, and thighs. By directing blood flow, the Reshape Program alone succeeds in depositing fat only where you want it. This fantastic result is naturally not achieved by exercise alone but by a combination of techniques. The special exercises performed in the correct way and at the right time, however, play a very important part in the lovely outcome.

Heat—Can Fat Be "Melted"?

One of the reasons why animals, including man, store energy in the form of fat is that fat is mostly liquid at body temperature, thus allowing for instant fat release in time of necessity. Not all components of body fat, however, are in fact liquid at body temperature (for instance, tripalmitin and tristearin are solid, although their interaction to some extent lowers their individual melting points), and since in order to move fat out of the fat cells it has to be in a liquid state, we must either (1) lower its melting point, or (2) raise our body temperature.

There is some evidence that unsaturated dietary fat may act to help body fat stay liquid, but apart from making sure that most of our fat intake is of the unsaturated kind, there's not much we can consciously do about lowering the melting point of something as unfamiliar to us as the isomers of our triglycerides (even though we may have been carrying them around on our hips for the past twenty years!). We can, however, raise the body temperature in selected areas in the following ways:

1. through friction, such as rubbing or massaging,
2. bathing the area in comfortably hot water, as in a hip bath,
3. applying hot compresses,
4. wearing the Reshape slimming pants,
5. applying an ointment to keep in body heat.

Heat also acts to dilate blood vessels, making it easier for blood to circulate freely.

Massage

Like "spot-reducing" exercises, massage will do nothing to actually make you lose weight. All the same, it has a very important role in the Woman's Reshape Program, for it helps to loosen and break up stubborn fat tissue exactly where you want to. Massage also locally raises the temperature, as we have seen. Also, it stimulates blood flow.

In the Reshape Program we employ both the Western type of massage—a combination of thumping, kneading, slapping, and so forth—and the Oriental type of finger pressure to stimulate the nervous system and in some cases possibly the hormonal flow. You'll find massage rewarding both as an outlet for your emotions, aimed directly at the object of your vexation—your fat bulges—and as a form of relaxation. If you have someone else to do some of the massaging for you, that's fine, but you can easily do it yourself all alone. In fact, the massage you do yourself helps to burn extra energy. As a bonus, it makes your fingers strong and supple, tightens the muscles in your arms and chest, and gives you the sensation of literally "shaping" your own body.

Perspiration

Fat cells contain not only fat but also waste products and water. In fact, those parts of the body that have excessive accumulations of female hormones, such as thighs and buttocks, tend to retain water even more than elsewhere. This is especially true if there's too much sodium (salt) in our body fluids, which is one good reason why we should cut down on salt. (Another reason is that salt, like any other strong condiment, irritates the stomach lining and therefore interferes with digestion.)

Accumulated fluid and waste, just like fat, causes the cells to swell and to bulge. Perspiring gets rid of a lot of the waste materials and, at least temporarily, some of the fluid—this being the basis for the claims of "lost three inches from hips and thighs in just twenty-five minutes" you often see in advertisements for slimming pants made of nonbreathing materials. Normally, the cells reabsorb the fluids again just as soon as a glass of water or other fluids are consumed. With the Reshape Program, however, you'll be able to at least partly prevent fluid from reaccumulating in the below-the-waist areas.

Should you already own one of these perspiration-inducing garments, then there's no reason why you shouldn't use it, provided you do so in accordance with the Reshape instructions. The Reshape sweat pants have several advantages, however: They're easy to slip on and off, they let your body "breathe" in the crotch, if you damage them you can replace them immediately (you have the necessary parts in your kitchen drawer), and they cost only a few cents.

Gravity

Animals, if they're obese, often have fat tummies, but you rarely see a nanny goat or a bitch with a fat rump or thick thighs. When Woman stood up on her hind legs, she brought down upon herself the curse of the law of gravity. But as is the case with most things, there are ways to make gravity work *for* us instead of against us, and Stage One of the Reshape Program will teach you how to do it.

Bandaging

In the course of our research, we came across a nineteenth-century family whose female members were famous for their slender ankles. (Those were the days when a quick glimpse of a trim feminine ankle would send male blood pressures soaring!) It was reported that from their earliest childhood, the girls of the family wound firm bandages around their ankles before they went to sleep.

Persistent strictures of this nature over long periods of time *will* prevent the deposition of fat in certain areas, but such methods would be most unpleasant and impractical, and also dangerous to health, especially where large areas such as hips, thighs, and buttocks are concerned. Who would want to go to sleep trussed like a mummy!

By being able to pinpoint the exact time (just a half hour or so) when fat-deposition would occur, and by combining it with other Reshape techniques employed at the same time, we succeeded in incorporating this very effective figure-shaping tool into our method in a way that is both safe and pleasant. And instead of unsightly bandages, a svelte pantie girdle will do the trick!

Biofeedback

That thirty minute lie-down some stunning women of the past used to enjoy before going to a ball or reception didn't merely serve them as physical rest—in the days of cooks and maids and nurses for the children, these women had precious little reason to feel tired—it was time used to *think themselves beautiful.* Modern research seems to confirm that through relaxed concentration we can in fact consciously influence so-called involuntary physiological functions, such as rate of heartbeat, or dilation and constriction of blood vessels. With the Reshape Program, the same kind of relaxed concentration Great-grandmother used instinctively to bring a rosy flush to her cheeks will help us direct rich blood flow to the area of our choice.

6

Lunch at Eliza's

A little over three years after our first tentative gropings toward our dream figures, twelve of the original sixteen creators of the Woman's Reshape Program gathered to wish me and my family bon voyage for our move to the United States. What a difference in all of us! We met for lunch at ultrachic Eliza's restaurant and drew admiring glances from the other guests and the kind of superattentive service from the waiters (a blasé lot!) that is normally reserved for food critics, celebrities, and Very Beautiful People. One of our young girls had indeed become a well-known model (not Sheree, though; she had married and was the mother of two babies but still retained her new slim figure), while the rest of us just looked like models and film stars. Some of us had less beautiful faces than others, some were not so young—but we had found that a slim, trim, and shapely figure is what people notice and admire most, and it is certainly what gives one the most self-confidence. We weren't just thin, we were terrific, and we knew it.

Let's Look at Some Great Results

At the beginning of our experiments we had each filled out a card stating weight, measurements, life-style, food fetishes, and any special problems. It had been my job to keep the records, and here are some of the original comments plus some final results.

PAULA   When we first started, Paula was forty-nine. She was 30 pounds over the desirable weight according to her life-insurance chart (much more lenient than our Reshape chart!), and she suffered from high blood pressure, exhaustion, and depression. "Has tried dozens of diets" her card reads, "but feels too sorry for herself to keep any of them up."

At our luncheon at Eliza's, Paula was one of the gayest and most talkative. She wore a green pantaloon suit only the slimmest of women can get away with, with an elegant filigree belt to emphasize her new small waist. Her chart shows that her weight had dropped from 151 pounds to 111 pounds, and her new measurements are: bust, 35 inches; waist, 24 inches; hips, 37 inches. "For me," she said to me as we were saying our good-byes, "life actually began at fifty."

URSULA   This tall, large-boned woman was the physical education teacher who had worked in health-and-beauty spas in Europe. Her overseas experiences in those luxury establishments had contributed a lot to our knowledge, yet she had previously been unable to do much about her own figure. Ursula was neither overweight nor flabby. In fact, her body was too muscular, with broad hips, a flat chest, and hard, angular lines.

Ursula's weight has barely changed. The reduction in her hips has been only two inches. But her bust increased by three full cup sizes, and her bones in the chest area have acquired a lovely feminine covering. Even her face looks softer, more womanly. Altogether, she has become a strikingly attractive woman.

GWENN   As a girl, Gwenn used to have a great figure. When she married, she started putting on weight. After two pregnancies, she weighed in at 138 pounds, which was 18 to 20 pounds above her single weight, and breast-feeding her babies had also caused her bustline to flop. Gwenn and her husband owned a nifty little yacht and spent their weekends on the blue waters of beautiful Sydney Harbor, where one of the inlets is famous for nude bathing. Gwenn used to watch her husband watch the nude beauties on the beach as they sailed by, and ate her heart out.

Today, Gwenn weighs 118 pounds. Her tummy is as flat as when she was a girl, and her bustline is almost as full and bouncy. Having known this couple for some years, I feel that her husband probably loved her just as much when she wasn't looking so terrific; but Gwenn was worried, she felt insecure, and a worried wife often steers toward troubled waters. So it is quite likely that by regaining her figure and her self-confidence, Gwenn actually saved her marriage.

LEANNE She was only nineteen when she already tipped the scales at 156 pounds. Her face was sallow and her hands and feet were always cold because she had such poor circulation. "Eats to compensate," Leanne's card was marked, "Favorite food: Italian pasta."

Leanne was one of our charter members, but she was unable to come to our luncheon, since she was in Fiji on a buying trip for the boutique she had recently opened in posh Double Bay (Sydney's equivalent of Rodeo Drive). She had come to my home to say good-bye before she left—a tall, slim, sensational-looking young career woman weighing 108 pounds and with a near-perfect (35-26-36) figure. I admired her vibrant good looks and she confessed, "I still eat when I have a problem." But instead of pasta, she now tucks into *főzelék!*

I could go on for pages and pages. Women who never wore shorts now wearing tiny bikinis . . . women who never felt pride in their appearance now getting admiring glances. Not only the thirty-seven women who were actually involved in the development of the technique benefited, but many of their friends or relatives who learned the technique over the telephone or even through the mail.

JUDY was one of the thirty-seven but her sister Anne lives an hour's flight away in Melbourne. "Our mother thought a fat baby is a healthy baby, so she fed us till we nearly burst,'' Judy once said. As a result, both girls had been fat and shapeless all their lives. They tried all kinds of diets, and sometimes managed to lose quite a lot of weight. Then their faces looked haggard, and instead of fat and shapeless, they looked just plain shapeless. Soon they put back all they had lost, anyway. "It wasn't worth the deprivation.''

Once Judy saw the improvements in her own figure, she passed the technique on to Anne in weekly letters, with little stick-figure illustrations for the exercises. According to Judy, the change in her sister is unbelievable, even more so than in herself, because on top of her other problems, Anne had also had a bad skin condition, which cleared up beautifully. This of course was due to better nutrition and better circulation.

Another out-of-town Reshaper was Margaret, who lives in Goulburn. She had heard about the method from a friend's friend and wrote to us for details. Six months later she sent a telegram: YOU'RE GENIUSES. BLESS YOU.

With the Reshape Program, you don't just lose weight, you self-create. Like a sculptor falling more and more in love with his creation, you mold and shape and taper yourself the figure of your dreams, and that gives you the will to persevere, and boosts you along with a sense of excitement and pride.

7

How to Calculate Your Ideal Weight and Your Desirable (Stupendous!) Measurements

Remember, we're aiming high. Our ideal measurements are based on those of some leading photographic models who must be extraslim to look great for the camera. So if you fall a little short of your aim, you'll still be pretty terrific!

Naturally, bone structure cannot be altered. There's nothing the Reshape Program can do about the underlying skeleton, nor can it greatly influence the amount of glandular tissue in the breasts, although some of the techniques are designed to stimulate glandular efficiency. But if you follow the Reshape Program with enthusiasm, then the stuff that covers the skeleton and the organs—muscle and fat—will be like sculptor's clay in your hands, to slim and to smoothe, to shape and to round as you please.

Just as a sculptor has a basic design when he starts building clay around his wire "skeleton," so you must also know exactly what dimensions you're aiming for. You already know how to calculate your ideal weight. Here's how to calculate your ideal measurements.

Wrist measurement in most people is pretty nearly matched to height. So once again we concentrate on the circumference of the wrists right on the wrist bone. You already know yours, for you probably checked it to make sure you're neither excessively small- nor excessively large-boned. In all probability you found your measurement between 6 inches and 6½ inches. Double that figure to get your ideal calf measurement, and triple it to get the correct circumference at midthigh. To this last figure, add two inches for the upper thigh, just beneath the buttock. Waist should be four times the wrist, hips and bust six times the wrist.

Let's say you're five feet six inches tall, twenty-five years old, and your wrists measure 6⅛ inches. Accordingly, your ideal vital statistics are:

WEIGHT:	First 5 feet of height	100 pounds
	3 pounds for each additional inch	+18
	Adjustment for age	− 0
	Adjustment, bone structure	− 0
	Ideal weight	118 pounds
MEASUREMENTS:	Wrist	6⅛ inches
	Calves (2 × wrist)	12¼ inches
	Mid thigh (3 × wrist)	18⅜ inches
	Upper thigh (3 × wrist + 2 inches) ...	20⅜ inches
	Waist (4 × wrist)	24½ inches
	Hips (6 × wrist)	36¾ inches
	Bust (6 × wrist)	36¾ inches

Now that's a fabulous figure even for a Miss Universe, and just as the judges of beauty contests allow some leeway, so do we, without sacrificing true figure beauty.

Range of Allowable Variation

In general, you can allow yourself a leeway of up to 1¼ inches at each point, but there should be no more than two inches of difference between the bust and the hips. In other words, the above figure with a *plus* of 1 inch at the thighs and/or hips and a 1¼ inch *minus* at the waist would still be pretty great, but if the bust is also 1¼ inches *minus* (35½ inches), then the hips should be no more than ¾ inches *plus* (37½ inches) to keep it within two inches of the bust.

How Often Should You Check Your Weight and Measurements?

Many reducing manuals advise checking weight only once a week, since daily weight fluctuations may be due to many factors other than true weight-loss or gain. Fluid retention is one such reason given. With the Reshape Method, however, we check our weight and our measurements *every morning*. Here's why.

While there's plenty of variety in the Reshape Diet, the quantity and the type of foods you eat are pretty nearly uniform, and so is the amount of liquid you drink. As long as you understand that a minor divergence in your weight or measurements is nothing to get excited about, the daily check will help to keep you on the straight and narrow, and besides, it's a thrill to see every day how well you're doing. Personally, I could hardly wait, and would check and recheck—and gloat!—several times even on the same morning. My weight and measurements are very stable now, but when I first started to reduce they used to fluctuate a little, and once I had reached my ideal goals (my ideal weight was, and is, 110 pounds), my hip measurement, which was my danger point, used to zigzag up to half an inch in either direction of 36 inches, and my weight up to three pounds between 109 and 112. When weight and measurement were at the low end of these permissible fluctuations, I relaxed and felt great. When they climbed to the upper limit, I knew I must be on the alert, and in fact managed to bring them back to target point within a couple of days, by simply adding another five minutes of running to my daily routine and cutting out such luxuries as sour cream or honey. Had I let them go beyond those narrow limits, then I would have had to work much harder to bring them down again, and who wants to go over ground already conquered? So the rule is: Check weight and measurements at the same time every morning, after you have emptied bowels and bladder, but before you've eaten, had anything to drink, or done many of the Reshape activities. Write down the results for daily comparison in any exercise book, but record on the Progress Recording Chart only every two weeks, when you must see real, substantial results.

How to Take Your Vital Statistics

WEIGHT

Weight, of course, must be taken without any clothes on. If you have an ordinary step-on bathroom scale, adjust it so that the indicator is smack on zero, then fix it in place by covering the adjusting wheel with tape. This is a *must*, or else you'll be fiddling with it all the time and never get the identical setting. Even with this precaution it is possible to make the needle go up or down a little by placing your weight unevenly; so make sure you stand on both feet square and fair, and don't cheat.

MEASUREMENTS

Always use the same tape measure and make sure you don't stretch it; we've had stretched tapes that differed from new ones by as much as three quarters of an inch. You won't stretch the tape if you take your measurements the correct Reshape way.

Stand in your bare feet before a mirror, without any clothes on. Taking the tape between forefinger and thumb, slide it gently around the area to be measured. Tape ends should barely touch, tape should slide easily over the skin. For measuring bust, waist, and hips, stand in the Reshape Posture.

THE RESHAPE POSTURE

This is the posture you will be practicing several times every day, until it becomes perfectly natural to you. It is also the posture best suited to taking your bust measurement.

Stand erect, head straight, shoulders dropped, stomach in, tail tucked under, head poised on your neck, as if an imaginary string attached to the top of your head were being gently pulled upward. Breathe normally.

Keeping your arms by your sides, bend your elbows and with both index fingers point to a spot about one inch above and out from the tip of each breast. Using the muscles that lie behind the upper part of each breast, and without moving your body, try to touch your breasts to your pointing fingers. Of course you can't actually make contact—the idea is to strain upward, lifting the breasts up and out. Once you've done this a few times, you'll be able to lift your chest toward imaginary "pointing fingers" without actually using your hands at all, and eventually the posture will become natural to you and contribute a great deal to the beauty of your figure.

Do remember, though, to let your shoulders drop to their normal position. Relax your shoulders, your head, and your neck. The "lifting" must be done entirely by the chest muscles. (See how it slims and streamlines your stomach!) Breathe normally throughout.

BUST

To measure your bust, hold the Reshape Posture, breathe normally, then hold your breath when you have partly *exhaled*. Your lungs will not be inflated, giving a false measurement, but your posture will be making the most of the shape you have. Since this posture will eventually be your normal one, that will be your "true" bust measurement.

Run the tape around the most prominent perimeter, but make sure the tape is straight all around. Remember, tape should be loose, slightly touching. You should be able to slide it around quite easily, but do not leave any slack.

WAIST

Maintain Reshape Posture. Do not hold your breath, breathe normally throughout.

TUMMY

This measurement does not figure on our Progress Recording Chart, but it is a useful one to chart your day-to-day general progress. Still maintaining the Reshape Posture, the tape held straight and slightly touching, measure around the prominence of hipbone about an inch under the navel.

HIPS

You must measure around the widest point of your derrière. The exact latitude varies from person to person. Find the right spot by looking in the mirror first full-face, then in profile. Double-check by letting the tape slide up and down your body. If it slides fairly easily over all the hip area (you may help a little with your free hand), then you know that the tape is recording the biggest measurement.

THIGHS AND CALVES

Stand about a foot away from the edge of bath or low stool. Place your right foot on the edge and measure first at midthigh, then at the highest point nearest the trunk. Next, measure the calf. Finally, step down, place your weight on your right foot, and measure the thigh again, around the widest part. As a rule, there's a difference of up to one inch—in the vertical position the thigh is that much thicker. The last measurement is again for your day-to-day progress checking only. For your vital statistics, you only need to record the thigh in the lifted positions, your foot resting on the edge of the bath or stool.

If you're like most people, one of your legs is probably a bit heavier than the other. You need not bother measuring the second leg daily, just make sure that whatever slimming activity you perform, always start with the heavier leg. Since one tends to be more vigorous at the beginning, the heavier leg will regularly come in for more effective treatment, and soon the difference between the two will disappear.

Your Weight and Measurement Progress Recording Chart

Using the calculations as set down on page 53, write in the appropriate places your desirable weight and all your target measurements. At the far left of your Progress Recording Chart, enter your weight and your measurements as they are today. Continue to record them every two weeks, and see how you're steadily nearing your fabulous model-girl proportions!

The Three Stages of the Woman's Total Reshape Program

The Reshape Program is divided into three distinct stages. Stage One is designed to trim off excess weight quickly and pleasantly, also to melt away inches and to begin firming and toning your body all over. In this section you'll become acquainted with all the basic elements of the Reshape Method, and establish a manner of eating you will want to enjoy the rest of your life. Read the section on Stage One, then put it aside—from then on, all you'll need is the handy, easy-to-follow Summary setting out step-by-step and day-by-day all you need to do.

When you have reached your *minimum* weight and measurements, you may go on to Stage Two—this will show you how to *maintain* your new light weight and slimness for all time, correct problems of posture and muscle development, and lay the foundations for your fabulous new bustline. Stage Three will balance your figure by lifting, firming, and adding lovely shapely inches to your breasts.

See Your Doctor

Before you undertake any diet or exercise program, it is wise to consult your own doctor. So be sure to have your personal physician check you out before you begin your Reshape Program.

Once you get your doctor's okay, go to it with enthusiasm, but don't let impatience make you reckless. If you're out of condition, if you haven't been doing any sport or strenuous exercise for ages, be sure to start slowly at first. Cut the recommended number of minutes or repetitions to one third at the beginning, and slowly work up to the full quota. If you do it gradually and persistently, a couple of weeks in low gear will probably be sufficient preparation. Let your personal physician be your guide.

Your Progress Recording Chart

AT THE BEGINNING OF THE RESHAPE PROGRAM

WRITE HERE YOUR HEIGHT:
YOUR WRIST MEASUREMENT:

AT THE END OF THE RESHAPE PROGRAM

WEIGHT										WEIGHT
BUST										BUST
WAIST										WAIST
HIP										HIP
THIGH										THIGH
CALF										CALF

RECORD YOUR PROGRESS ON THIS CHART
ONLY ONCE EVERY TWO WEEKS.

In the far left column, enter your weight and your measurements as they are today, at the beginning of the Reshape Program. Taking your height and your wrist measurement as your guides, work out your ideal weight and your desirable measurements according to the directions on pages 27 and 53. Enter them in the far right column RIGHT NOW—and start watching that dream becoming a reality! Every two weeks, you'll note how you're getting closer and closer to your ideal figure.

PART II

The Woman's Total Reshape Program—

Stage One

LOSE WEIGHT AND INCHES ALL OVER
QUICKLY AND PLEASANTLY
(WITH SPECIAL ATTENTION
TO WAIST, HIPS, AND THIGHS).

8

The Reshape Activities

Nnone of us thirty-seven lazy ladies actually liked to exercise, so exercises have been kept to a minimum in the Reshape Program and planned in such small doses that they're never tiring or boring. The little exercise we do, however, must be done not only at the right time, but also in the right way, to yield the most good.

Learn How to Breathe

If you want to lift a heavy object, you instinctively take a deep breath and hold it while you do the lifting. The same should be true of any exercise. You take in air when you're directing your muscles to do some work, and you let the air out when you allow your muscles to relax.

Place the tips of your fingers vertically just above your waist. Take a deep, slow breath through your nose, until the fingertips of your two hands are lifted *apart*. Hold it to a count of three, then let the breath out through your mouth. Do this a few times, breathing in s-l-o-w-l-y through the nose—hold 1-2-3—out through the mouth. Now do the same thing while you're lifting your left knee. Breathe *in* as the leg comes up—hold—breathe *out* as the leg goes down and the muscles relax. Repeat with the other knee. Now do the same thing *faster*—the important thing is to remember that you breathe *in* when you're causing your muscles to tense, and you breathe *out* when you're telling them to relax.

Stretch Your Limits—Slowly

When you're doing the exercises, remember to stretch the muscles only to the point where you *begin* to feel discomfort, no further. Stop, then repeat. On experiencing discomfort, stop again, then repeat. Each time you repeat, your point of discomfort will move back a little further, until you're able to do your maximum with ease.

The In-Bed Routine

Your Reshape day begins as soon as you open your eyes in the morning—in the comfort of your bed.

During sleep, blood tends to collect around the internal organs, leaving the peripheral areas, including the brain, with decreased circulation. That is the reason why we sometimes feel woozy or dizzy when we first jump out of bed. The following in-bed exercises will redistribute the blood supply, make you wide-awake and full of pep.

Start with only a few of each exercise; work up to the prescribed numbers over the next few days.

1. The Stretch

Lying comfortably on your back, stretch slowly and luxuriously, yawn, tense all your muscles in turn; flex your ankles, bend your feet up and back . . . down . . . up and back . . . down; rotate your ankles, feet describing outward circles . . . then inward circles.

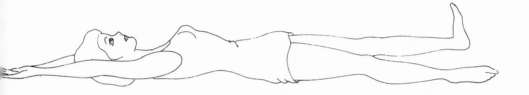

The following leg movements should be done with a smooth, flowing rhythm, without pausing between them, and without your heels coming to rest on the bed.

2. The Vertical Leg-Lift

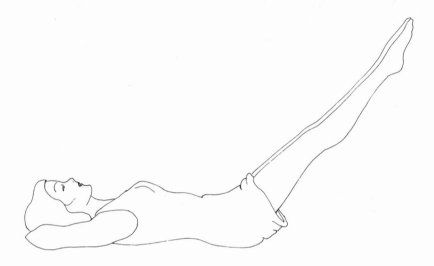

Interlace your fingers behind your neck. Feet together, knees straight, toes pointing, raise your legs until they're almost, but not quite, vertical, then lower them to within a couple of inches from the bed. Repeat up to ten times, then, without pausing, go into—

3. The Knees-to-Chest

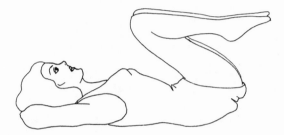

Bend both knees to chest, then straighten them to horizontal, keeping your heels from touching the bed. Do this up to ten times, then—

4. The Scissors

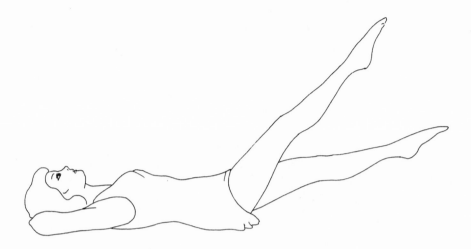

Heels off the sheet, lift alternate legs up to ten times in a fast, vertical scissors movement.

Relax. Lift your pelvis off the bed and shake, to help relax your muscles. Rest for a few seconds.

5. The Isometric Ankle-Cross

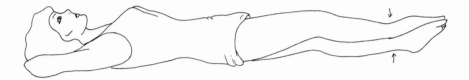

Still keeping your hands behind the back of your neck, cross your ankles and press top leg downward against bottom leg, while bottom leg presses upward, offering resistance. Hold to a count of six. Repeat with legs reversed.

6. Isometric Wrist-Push and Wrist-Pull

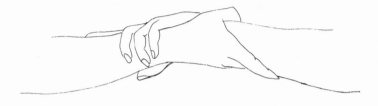

Grabbing wrists of opposite hands, try to push together ten times. Then push, and hold to a count of six. Now try to pull apart ten times, then pull, and hold to a count of six.

Relax.

The entire in-bed routine should take you no more than five minutes. Apart from getting you off to a vibrant start, these exercises provide an easy minimum-maintenance routine in case you ever need to miss out on the rest of the day's exercise activities. Having them behind you, you won't spend the rest of the day feeling so flabby nor so guilty! So skip something else if you absolutely cannot spare the time, but never skip your in-bed routine!

Let's Mobilize—The Reshape Way!

The nutrients in the last meal you ate at about 6 or 7 P.M. the previous night have been fully digested and absorbed. Their amino acids have gone to repair or build new body structures, their vitamins, minerals, and other components have been used up in the process of assimilation. Their calories in the form of glucose have been burned up to create energy. The small amount of glucose still in your bloodstream and the glycogen stored in your liver are sufficient to provide the brain and the nervous system with their needs. Should there be a sudden increased demand for energy, your body will have no choice but to go to work recruiting energy by converting fat from your fat stores. This is why the bulk of the Reshape activities are done in the morning before you have had anything to eat or to drink; your blood glucose levels are low, your insulin levels are low, the conditions are perfect for the mobilization of fat from your hard-to-budge bulk fat depots.

The combination of activities that follow will alternately call for increased energy supplies, soften and break down stubborn fat deposits to free them into the bloodstream, and prevent circulating fat from resettling in its favorite areas.

Stretching and Firming

Do the following routines in your bedroom or in any room where you have privacy, and where you can have the window open to allow plenty of fresh air. If possible, wear nothing—this will allow your skin to take an air bath while you work out.

Concentrate on what you are doing, and *enjoy* your movements. Be conscious of each area of muscles as you work them. It's a great feeling to get in touch with your body!

1. The Reach for the Ceiling

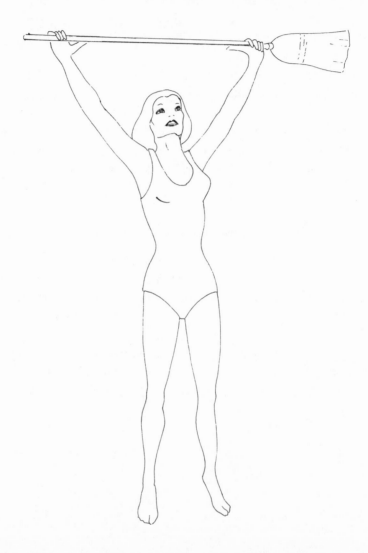

Grab a broom handle in both hands. Stand up straight, and stretch as if you were trying to reach the ceiling.

2. The Side Twist

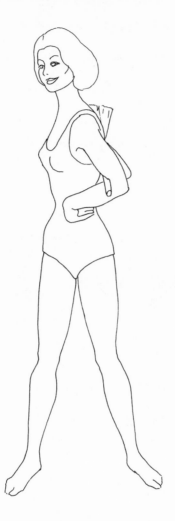

Holding the broom handle in the crooks of your arms behind your back, legs slightly apart and feet pointing straight ahead, turn from waist as far as you can without moving the hips too, and do two bumps to the right . . . then turn in the opposite direction and do two bumps to the left. Repeat ten times. Then, swinging hard, do single bumps right, left, right, left, ten times.

3. The Side Bend

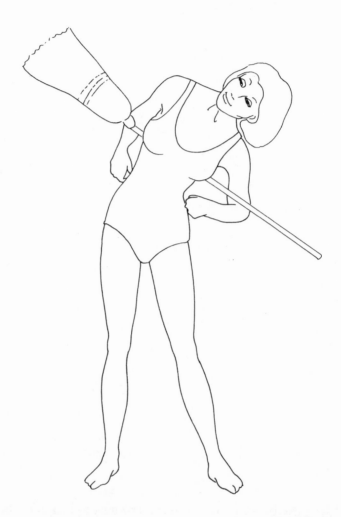

Again using the double bump, broom handle behind your back in the crooks of your arms, bend to the right—bump, bump—then to the left—bump, bump—ten times. Then swinging really hard, do single bumps in each direction, right, left, right, left, ten times.

4. The Backward and Forward Bend

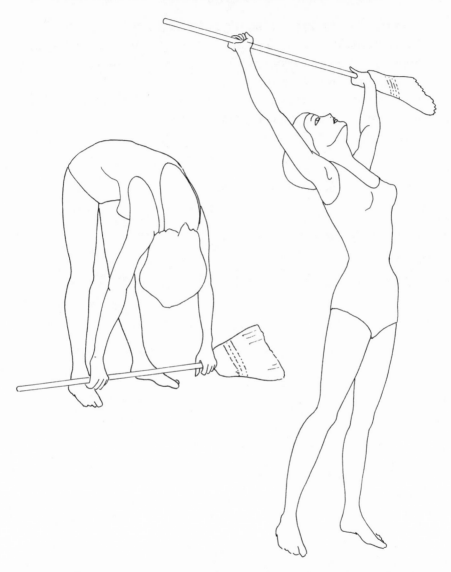

Using the double bump as before, and stretching upward with the broom held in both hands, bend backward as far as you can—bump, bump—then forward, touching the broom to the floor if you can—bump, bump—ten times. Then swinging hard again, do ten combined backward-and-forward bends.

FIRST HARD CALL FOR ENERGY

Put aside the broom, stand up straight and jump rhythmically, spreading your feet and clapping your palms together
above your head as you rise into the air on the first jump, then
bringing feet together and arms down by your side on the next.
Keep jumping up to twenty-five times, breathing in as you raise
your arms, out as you bring them down.

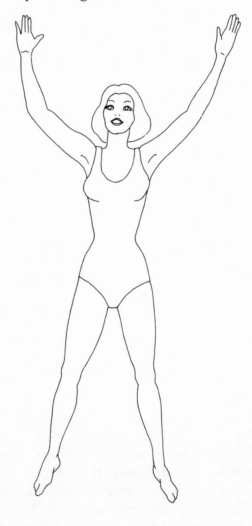

Increased energy need (fat-burning) goes on for several minutes after you stop the exercise; during these important minutes, you'll be liberating unwanted bulk fat into the bloodstream through massage.

Massage

You'll be employing five varieties of massage: hand massage, floor massage, friction massage, wall massage, and broom-handle massage. Always massage carefully, never hard enough to bruise.

HAND MASSAGE

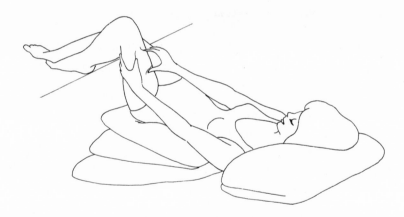

Place three pillows or three thickly folded blankets on the floor close to the end of your bed, and one single pillow next to them. Position yourself so that your head and shoulders rest on the single pillow, your hips and buttocks higher, on the three pillows or folded blankets, and your legs and feet the highest, on the bed. All your movements will be *downward, toward the heart.*

Before beginning the actual massage, stimulate the nerve ends by using finger pressure on your feet and ankles.

FINGER PRESSURE

Starting with the heavier leg, grab your foot with both hands and rotate it a few times in each direction. Then grab your big toe between thumb and index finger, and rotate toe a few times to the right and to the left. Repeat with each toe in turn. Supporting your foot with your other hand, gently massage with your thumb in a rotating movement the top of your foot just above the line of your toes. This is a wonderfully sensuous feeling, and in fact is said to stimulate the glands of the breasts. Next, massage the whole foot, applying pressure gently with the balls of your fingers. Don't forget the insteps and the base of the toes. Finally, press between thumb and forefinger, at about one-inch intervals all around the heel and along the muscle at the back of the ankle. Proceed to leg massage.

The four elements of massage by hand are:

1. *Gentle stroking.* With the flats of all the fingers of both hands, gently stroke downward (remember, you're upside down), *toward the heart.*

2. *Kneading.* This is more vigorous (but gentle enough never to cause pain or bruising!), using both hands as if you were kneading dough. Dig in with your knuckles; grab the roll of fat with both hands and move it around in opposite directions; squeeze it, wring it.

3. *Scoring.* Imagine that you have dislodged fat and waste material from the tissues, and want to drive them toward the trunk where vigorous circulation will carry them away. To do this, stroke hard with the straight edge of your hands, or with the bent knuckles of all the fingers in a "scoring" manner, always in the direction of the heart.

4. *Slapping.* To finish, slap the whole area with the open palms of both hands.

You start the massage at the ankle and work up to the knee (not forgetting the inside of the knee!), the midthigh, and the inside and the outer bulge at the top of the thigh.

Work on one leg at a time, alternately

- Stroking with the flats of your fingers
- Gently pinching with the tips of your fingers
- Squeezing large chunks with the whole hand
- Wringing with both hands
- Scoring with knuckles or edge of hand
- Slapping with open palms.

To work on the hips and the buttocks, turn on one side: use one hand at a time.

SECOND HARD CALL FOR ENERGY

When hand massage is finished, stand up, and do ten vigorous knee-bends to direct maximum blood flow to the hip and leg area, and to cause renewed fat-burning by the additional call for energy.

Now drop back on the pillows, hips and buttocks raised, legs resting on the bed, and relax for a couple of minutes, letting gravity carry the freshly released fat in the blood stream *away* from the fat-prone area.

FLOOR MASSAGE

This is powerful massage, where you let the floor do most of the work. If your bedroom carpet is too thick and soft, do it in the bathroom and use a rug.

1. The Side Roll

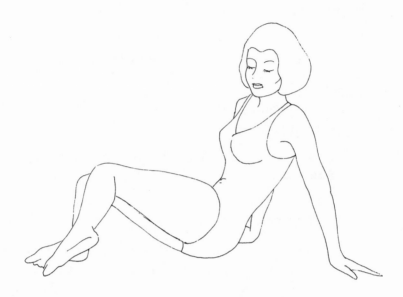

Sitting on the floor, with knees half-bent, roll from side to side, pressing buttocks to the floor. You can vary the area being massaged by leaning back on your elbows or lying back on the floor, letting your hips get most of the action.

2. The Side Rock

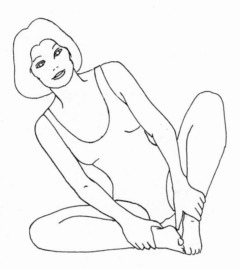

Sitting up, knees apart, feet together and close to your body, hold ankles and roll from side to side.

3. The Fanny Press

Sitting up again, knees bent, soles resting on the floor, press the soft tissue of your buttocks against the floor and move backward and forward *inside your skin*.

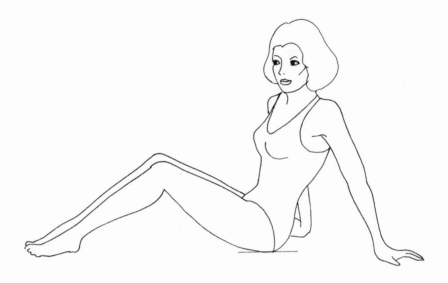

Do each of the above up to twenty-five times. When you have finished, support your hips on your hands and, resting your head comfortably on the single pillow, do ten bicycle kicks in the air. Then leave your hips and legs elevated on the pillows and bed, and relax.

Your Reshape activities so far—in-bed exercises, stretching and firming exercises, hand massage, floor massage—have taken a total of about twenty-five to thirty minutes. If you can afford the time, and if you want your progress to be rapid, then you must go on to the friction-massage and the slimming pants and include them in your routine every day, at least for the first few weeks. If you absolutely cannot spare the time during the week, then do these only on the weekends. (However, you *must* do your five- to ten-minute run *every morning*. If you must skip the friction rub and the slimming pants, then slip into a pair of warm-up pants and cotton blouse and go directly to the section on "Hard Call for Energy.")

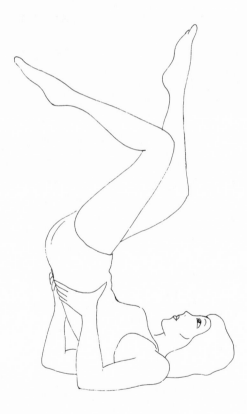

FRICTION MASSAGE

Turn on the taps in your bath (if there's no tub in your bathroom, the hot shower will do), and while it is filling to hip-level with *comfortably* hot water, weigh yourself and take your measurements as explained earlier, and as set out in the Summary. If the results are less than thrilling, promise yourself an extra two minutes running. If they're great, you're allowed a quick gloat in the mirror.

Lower yourself into the hip-bath, which is just pleasantly hot (we want to *melt* the fat, not fry it!), and with a loofah or rough washcloth, friction-rub with firm, circular movements your thighs, buttocks, and abdomen until the skin is a healthy pink color.

Quickly pat yourself dry and slip on your Reshape slimming pants.

Your Seventeen-Cent Replaceable Slimming Pants

There are various perspiration-inducing gadgets on the market, from portable home saunas to airtight plastic pants, and if you already own a pair of the latter, then there's no reason why you shouldn't use it instead of the Reshape pants. All the same, we found that apart from being costly and not very durable, these airtight pants have some other drawbacks: the tight-fitting variety is very hard to put on and even harder to take off, while the loose type that depends on a suction machine to suck the air out keeps you fixed to the spot. Both types keep you completely airtight from waist to knees and both types need to be completely removed in case you want to use the bathroom.

The Reshape slimming pants cost practically nothing, their parts can be replaced if damaged, they're easy to put on and to take off, they do not curtail your mobility, and they allow air to the crotch area. They're simply a trio of plastic bags, such as you use in your kitchen garbage can!

Use bag size two feet by two feet 6 inches (tall kitchen bag size). Cut open at bottom ends. Slip one bag over your legs and up to just below the bust and hold it in place by tying a ribbon or cord around the waist. Pull a pair of stretch briefs over the plastic bag, making sure that the bottom ends of the bag extend downward over your thighs. Pull the other two bags over each leg, tuck them into the briefs at the top. Holding the lower ends to the knees, pull a pair of old ballet tights or old pantyhose (anything tight enough to hold the plastic close to your body) over the whole thing (in hot weather, I cut off the feet of the

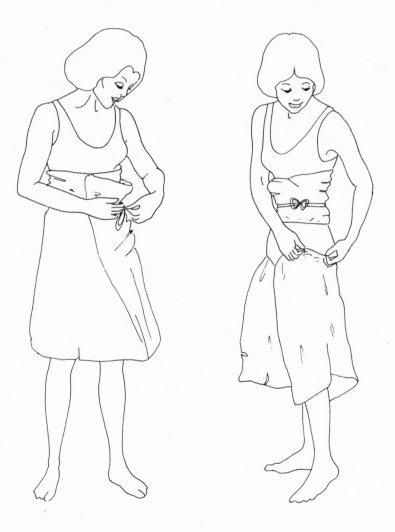

tights to allow ventilation), and that's all. If above waist and midriff need reducing, tie a stretchy scarf around those areas, or slip on an elasticized tank top (not over the breasts!) or hold the plastic in place, *under* your bosom, with a length of elastic bandages.

For added warmth, pull on a pair of fleecy warm-up pants; on the top part of your torso wear a cotton vest or a cool cotton blouse.

THIRD, EXTRAHARD CALL FOR ENERGY

Your bulk fat depots have had a thorough shake-up; you've loosened them through different kinds of massage, you've melted them with heat from water and from friction, and right now they're being worked on by your slimming pants. Now they're more than ready to move out—all you need is for your body to call for an extralarge shot of energy.

Remember, the biggest muscles need the most energy, and the biggest muscles are in the legs and buttocks, so the quickest way to call for large stores of energy is to *run, skip,* or *jump.* You may jog around the living room, you may skip in place on the balcony, or you can jump rope—the important thing is to lift your feet at least six inches off the ground and really *move.* Turn on your oven timer or an alarm clock and starting with two minutes, work up to five, and eventually to ten minutes. Slow down from time to time if you must, but every now and again be sure to burst into a really vigorous sprint. One great energy-gobbler is a fast gallop every now and again just the way you used to do when you were a kid pretending that you were riding a horse. Holding your hands in front of you as if you were gripping reins, lift yourself with every "hoof" beat as if you were rising in the saddle. This is terrific exercise and it gives you a great "high."

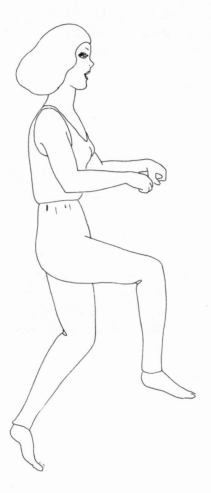

WHEN YOU STOP . . .

Blood is racing to and from the big muscle areas in your thighs and buttocks. Along with oxygen and other nutrients, this blood contains fat particles freshly released from your fat depots. When you stop running, the effect of gravity will tend to keep the greater part of this fat-rich blood in the lower portion of your body, causing light-headedness, and resulting in a great deal of the circulating fat resettling in the fat-prone areas all over again. To avoid these effects, as soon as your timer buzzes, lie down on a couch or on the floor and stay horizontal until your breathing has returned to normal. At this stage the fat-rich blood is still cruising in your veins, so you must adopt a position to counteract gravity.

THE RESHAPE ANTIGRAVITY POSITION

You really need something a little steeper than the fifteen-inch-or-so incline of the ordinary slant board. If you happen to own a slant board, you can prop the high end on something that will add an extra few inches. But you are really much better off using an ordinary armchair. Here's how to do it.

Stand facing the side of an upholstered armchair. Lean over the armrest and place both hands on the front of the seat. Bring your knees up on the armrest, slide forward, and placing your palms on the floor in front of the chair, swing your legs up and rest your feet over the back of the chair. It may sound tricky, but it is really very easy to do and it works much better than a slant board because the incline is much steeper, and there is no pressure on your breasts while they benefit fully from the pull of gravity. Also, it costs nothing, and you don't need to bother setting up or having to store a clumsy 6-foot board.

Remain in the antigravity position for as long as you feel comfortable. You may change the position of your arms or your head as you get tired, or you may even lie on the floor for a while, then return to the antigravity position for another spell. Relax—listen to music, daydream, plan your new wardrobe!

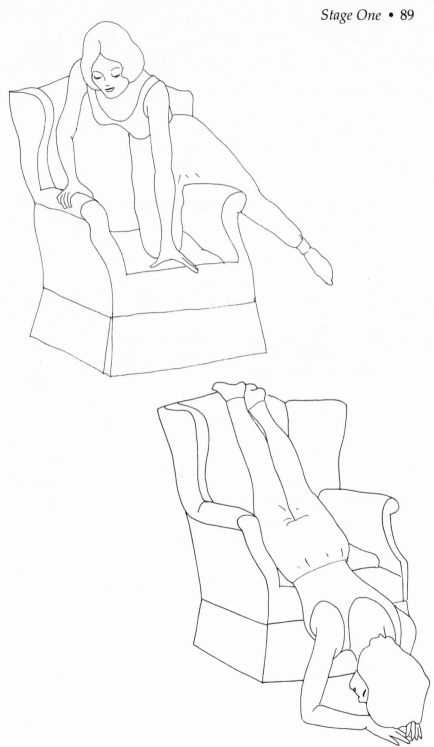

MEANWHILE, YOUR SLIMMING PANTS ARE WORKING

While the foregoing was happening, your slimming pants were removing accumulated wastes through the pores, as well as a great deal of fluid. Under ordinary conditions, the resulting weight-loss and inch-loss would only be very temporary, as a couple of glasses of water quickly restore what has been lost (or rather, make you lose again what you have gained!); in fact, on its own, perspiring will not achieve lasting results. As part of the overall Reshape Program, however, it contributes a great deal, especially in the beginning. That's why in the first few weeks, you should try to do the *complete* Reshape Program every day, particularly if you have the kind of solid bulk fat on hips and thighs that benefits enormously from every type of softening and liquefying you can give it. Once you have loosened this kind of tissue and shed a few pounds from the area, you may skip the hot friction massage and the slimming pants. But of course you must return to them every once in a while, say once or twice every week or every two weeks.

But for the moment, let's go back to where we left off—upside down on an armchair.

When you have relaxed in the antigravity position, rest *horizontally* for a minute or so to allow your circulation to normalize. Then get up and go about your business making beds, preparing breakfast, or whatever you do at this time of the morning, keeping your slimming pants on while you work. Wear them also while you are performing a couple of additional massaging techniques. Since these are done against very hard surfaces, such as a solid wall and a sturdy broom handle, the layers of plastic and clothing you're wearing will give you needed protection.

WALL MASSAGE

This massage is especially for those who have what is often called "riding breeches"—those ugly bulging rolls of fat at the top of the thighs.

Stand against a solid wall and gently but firmly bump the bulging part of your thigh against it. Start with ten bumps and in a few days work up to one hundred quick bumps on each thigh.

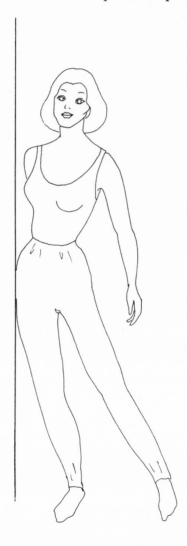

BROOM-HANDLE MASSAGE

Grab the broom handle in both hands and gently but firmly work it backward and forward on any bulge area: the "riding breeches," the insides of the thighs, the inside of the knees, the buttocks.

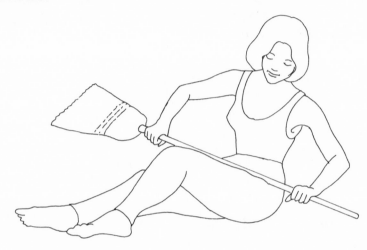

IMPORTANT: Follow with some vigorous pats with the palms of your hands, then do a quick burst of bicycling in the air. Stay for a minute or so in the upside-down position, legs pointing toward the ceiling, to allow the blood to flow back.

You may keep your slimming pants on for as little or as long as you like. When you've taken them off, wipe them clean with a wet cloth, dry them, and fold them, storing them in reverse order so that you will be able to put them on again quickly tomorrow: warm-up pants on the bottom, then the pantyhose, next the two plastic bags for the legs, next the stretch briefs, then the ribbon for the waist, and finally bag number one. You'll save time and induce perspiration quicker if you can put them on as soon as you've stepped from your hot hip-bath.

After a cool shower, spread oil or cream over your problem areas. The thin film will help to retain body heat as well as restore suppleness to the skin where water and the salt in perspiration may have dried it out.

9

The Reshape Diet

It's Time for a Drink!

Here's to your health—and beauty. Nothing more bracing, though, than a tall glass of sparkling fresh water.

You've taken off your slimming pants and enjoyed a cool shower. All your Reshape activities together took about one hour. You're pretty tired but you feel invigorated, and you're more thirsty than you're hungry. Propped up on your elbow on your bed or a sofa, or in warm weather on a sun-lounge on your balcony, slowly sip a large glass of water to which, if you like, the juice of a lemon has been added. If you can spare the time, stay horizontal for a few minutes to prevent the water from collecting in the tissues below the waist, which your slimming pants have just now freed from excess fluid. That's it—your concentrated Reshape activites are over for the day.

To Breakfast or Not to Break Fast?

Whether you now have breakfast or not is entirely up to you. Many of us found that it was easier to go through part of the day without taking any food at all, for once the "fast" is broken, one tends to crave more food. During the course of the morning, you'll be drinking another two or three glasses of water, which will have the effect of filling you up, and also give you some oral satisfaction. So if you choose not to have breakfast, then have a glass of water (warm, if you prefer) every time you feel you want to eat. Better still, do a few fast laps around the living room, or some leg bends, or other big-muscle exercise first and then have a glass of water, always sipping slowly and, if possible, in a horizontal position with the legs raised.

If you feel the need for eating breakfast, or if your doctor recommends that you do, there's absolutely no reason why you should not enjoy a poached egg or some cottage cheese, a piece of toast, a small glass of orange juice or some stewed fruit. For a rich taste, add a sprinkle of cinnamon to the fruit.

Nutrition: Make Every Calorie Count

If you're a woman of average height, your daily calorie allowance is in the 800- to 950-calorie range. You must stick to that. The important thing is to do the most you can with the permitted calories to avoid feeling miserable and deprived, while avoiding resorting to synthetic nonfoods. Let me stress once again: Our findings convinced us beyond any doubt that on a low-calorie diet, the more natural and nutritious the food, the quicker the weight-loss. The reason for this is really not hard to understand: The better the tools for the body to work with, the more efficient its metabolism. And when the bulk of your food intake consists of high-fiber, high-water, low-calorie, low-carbohydrate elements such as in the Reshape Diet, then you can have *real* honey (never sugar!), *real* oil dressing, *real* mayonnaise, even *real whipped cream* and still stay within the limits of your permitted calories. In Stage One you'll eat like a gourmet princess, in Stage Two you'll eat like a hearty queen, and in Stage Three you'll have a ball!

Some of the dishes in the recipes may be prepared beforehand and enjoyed cold, so if you have to pack a lunch, whether to take to work or a picnic, why not take a generous bowlful of luscious green bean *fözelék* in a container, and enjoy it with a cold chicken leg and a couple of crackers, plus a crisp, shiny apple.

If your height permits you to consume more calories than contained in the recipes, or if you find that you're losing too much weight too fast (the old two-pounds-a-week weight-loss is the safest), then adjust your food intake by adding extra protein (more fish or poultry, or you may substitute lean meat for these) and fruit. Do not increase the amount of the vegetables, as two pounds a day is quite enough, and certainly do not increase the quantity of oil and sour cream.

Simple Structure of the Reshape Diet

There are hundreds of different diets on the market. Much thought and research has gone into most, and apart from those that advocate lopsided nutrition that is in opposition to nature's requirements, many fill the bill quite adequately, though often they are a little too complicated. Since the Reshape Method, being a total figure-beautifying technique and not merely a weight-loss regime, has so many important elements other than diet, we have tried to keep the structure of the Reshape Diet simplicity itself, even though its components are as intricately delicious as any, and more satisfying than most.

Since for nutritional balance we need proteins, carbohydrates, vitamins, and minerals, and since these nutrients are preferably to be taken from meat, fish, and poultry, milk products, fruits, vegetables, and small amounts of fats (mostly in the form of unsaturated oils) and grains, the following is the simple basic structure of the Reshape Diet.

ON THE LOWEST (800 CALORIES) CALORIE REGIME, EACH DAY YOU WILL HAVE, APPROXIMATELY:

		Calories
3	ounces poultry or fish	120
1	small egg	70
3	ounces cottage cheese (½ percent butter fat)	60
1½	tablespoons oil* or butter	180
1½	pounds cooking vegetables plus ½ pound raw	150
1	tablespoon flour	25
1	tablespoon sour cream or whipped cream	40
1	slice whole wheat bread or cereal	55
Fruits		100
Total:		800

Naturally, if there's anything on this list you absolutely hate, or are medically warned against because of some allergy, there's no reason why you could not substitute some other item, as long as it is in the same category nutritionally, and as long as it contains no more calories. You may substitute more cottage cheese, or more fish or poultry for the egg, or you may exchange the cottage cheese for solid cheese (no more than 1 ounce!).

But basically, all the above are nutritional necessities, with the exception of the flour and the sour cream; the latter, however, are what separates the happy Reshape dieter from the ordinary, wretched variety!

Those Big, Delicious Meals—What to Have and How to Prepare Them

If you decided on having breakfast, then here's a breakup of the day's calorie intake:

	Calories
Breakfast	175
Lunch	200
Dinner	425
TOTAL:	800

*Use sesame or safflower oil, preferably cold-pressed.

BREAKFAST

The most nutritious and practical manner in which we may spend our 175 calories for this meal are small portions each of a cereal food, a protein food, and a fruit. Here are a few suggestions:

	Calories
⅔ cup unsweetened cereal (flakes or puffed)	50
⅔ cup skim milk, buttermilk, or ½ cup yogurt	60
Small portion of stewed fruit	65
TOTAL:	175

or

	Calories
Pancake made of 1 small egg	70
1½ teaspoon flour	10
¼ cup skim milk	20
½ small apple, thinly sliced	25
(Cook in nonstick pan and sprinkle with cinnamon)	
¾ cup strawberries or 1 medium peach	50
TOTAL:	175

or

	Calories
Medium tomato stuffed with 2 ounces cottage cheese	70
Topped with slivers (¼ ounce) of Cheddar or mozzarella	30
(Place under broiler till cheese melts)	
1 slice whole wheat bread	55
Pat of butter	20
TOTAL:	175

or

	Calories
½ of one chapati (thin, round unleavened bread from health-food store)	60
1 ounce cottage cheese spread over chapati	20
½ ounce slivered Cheddar or mozzarella	50
(Broil until cheese is melted, then roll up or fold like pancake)	
1 cup strawberries or two apricots	45
TOTAL:	175

(SUGGESTION: If you don't eat breakfast, shift the fruit to lunchtime for dessert; increase your dinnertime protein by about 70 calories—a second helping of fish or chicken—and use the bread at dinnertime to mop up the delicious *Gemüse* sauce!)

LUNCH

Here's the basic, nutritious menu structure for the midday meal:

	Calories
½ pound vegetables for soup or "hot salad"	50
Cottage cheese or equivalent	60
½ tablespoon oil or butter	60
Crackers or other	30
TOTAL:	200

DINNER

Your 425-calorie dinner is calculated on the basis of 3 ounces of poultry or fish, served with a brimful of rich-tasting vegetable *Gemüse* or *főzelék* and dessert. If chicken or fish is not your favorite food but steak is, then you may substitute steak or hamburger, lean meat broiled without added fat, and halve the *Gemüse.* It will still be a fairly substantial meal, though nowhere near as generous. The makeup of the menu is as follows:

	If protein food is fish or chicken	*If protein food is steak*
Protein food	120 Calories	245 Calories
Gemüse	255 Calories	130 Calories
Fruit dessert	50 Calories	50 Calories
TOTAL:	425	425

SOME HINTS ON PREPARING VEGETABLES FOR THE
RESHAPE RECIPES

Never soak vegetables, as this leeches out valuable nutrients, which will be lost in the water. Wash vegetables thoroughly in cold water, rinsing well under the tap. Carrots, asparagus, and celery stalks should be carefully scrubbed with a soft brush.

After you've cleaned the vegetables, cut off the tougher parts, but do not discard them at once. Instead, chop them up and simmer them for ten minutes in a cupful of gently boiling water. Strain cooking water into a cup, add a bouillon cube or a spoonful of high-protein vegetable extract, sprinkle with minced parsley or dill, and you have a delicious broth full of extra nutrients. Enjoy it as a first course at lunch or at dinner.

In the recipes that follow, calculations are based on edible portions, in the raw state. One pound of asparagus means one pound measured raw, *after* the tough parts have been cut off.

Half a pound of carrots means just that: half a pound of scraped, cleaned, ready-to-use vegetables with nothing to be thrown away. Place a large empty plate on your kitchen scales, adjust to zero, then keep trimming, washing, and scraping your vegetables and piling them onto the plate until you've reached the desired weight. Then proceed to cook them.

Some vegetables are over 100 calories per pound, others are under, as you can see on the Calorie Table which follows. Try to use them in combinations so that they even themselves out. However, it is understood that we burn more calories digesting vegetables than the calories they actually contribute (this is especially true of raw salad vegetables; that's why on most diets, including the Reshape Diet, they are "free"), so you really need not worry: As long as you use vegetables as your main bulk food (excepting, of course, the starchy ones such as corn and potato) and observe the limits on the *other* foods, the pounds will just melt away!

APPROXIMATE CALORIE TABLE FOR
ONE POUND OF VEGETABLES
(Fresh, raw, edible portions only)

	Calories
Asparagus	120
Beans, green	180
Beet greens	110
Broccoli	140
Brussels sprouts	200
Cabbage, Chinese	62
Cabbage, red	130
Cabbage, white	98
Cabbage, savoy	98
Carrot	190
Cauliflower	120
Celery	80
Chard, Swiss	110
Collards	180
Cress	130
Cucumber	70
Eggplant	110
Endive	90
Fennel	120
Kohlrabi	130
Leek	200
Lettuce	65
Mushroom	120
Mustard greens	130
Okra	160
Peas, young green	300
Pepper, green	100
Pepper, red	130
Pumpkin	120
Radish	85
Spinach	110
Tomato	90
Zucchini	80

SOME SUGGESTIONS FOR PREPARING MEAT, POULTRY, AND FISH

Chicken thighs or drumsticks Remove skin and fat. Place in vegetable steamer over gently boiling water. Cover with slices of tomato, salt, onion rings, herbs. Steam until tender.

Chicken breast Steam and cut up. Mix ¼ cup buttermilk, salt, and chives, add chicken chunks and simmer ten minutes.

Or, marinate in bouillon with tomato, garlic, onion, and herbs, then broil each side for fifteen minutes.

Ground veal Mix ground veal with salt and herbs, form into balls. Brown in nonstick skillet. Cover with bouillon, simmer for fifteen minutes.

Veal chops Sear in nonstick skillet. When brown, add some bouillon, onion, garlic, simmer till tender.

Liver Remove all veins, cut in strips. Drop into nonstick skillet and keep turning at very high heat until all sides are well seared. Add a little hot bouillon and chopped parsley. Turn down heat and simmer for a minute, until liver is cooked through. Salt and serve at once.

Fish fillets Bake or poach in a little of any of the cream soups.
Or, simmer in mixture of buttermilk, lemon juice, salt, cumin seeds, green pepper.
Or, mix cottage cheese, chives, spread on fish, broil for fifteen minutes.
Or, for a cold fish dish, bring to boil onion, salt, lemon juice, cold water. Add fish, simmer until cooked. Take out the fish, allow to cool. Pour liquid over fish, chill.

For dinner, serve the poultry, fish or meat alongside any of the rich vegetable dishes. Together, they should add up to no more than 375 calories.

APPROXIMATE CALORIE TABLE FOR 3½ OUNCES OF POULTRY, FISH OR MEAT
(Raw, edible portions only)

POULTRY: Calories
Chicken meat, dark 130
Chicken meat, light 125
Chicken giblets 140

FISH:
Abalone 110
Bass, sea or black 100
Carp 100
Catfish 100
Crab 100
Flounder 70
Kingfish 85
Lobster 90
Mussels 100
Oysters 100
Scallops 85
Shrimp 90
Sole 85
Trout 100

MEAT:
Beef heart 110
Beef kidney 150
Round steak 200
Club steak 300
Sirloin steak 250
Tongue 210
Liver 140
Ham, boiled 280
Veal chops 180

All values are for raw, edible portions only, with all visible fat cut off. In the case of chicken, two small drumsticks or one small leg is about three ounces. If in doubt, weigh the piece raw, then after cooking, remove and weigh the bone. The difference is the weight of the meat.

A WORD ABOUT DESSERT

There's no better way to finish a meal than with a perfect piece of sun-ripened fresh fruit. Cooking, mashing, grating, freezing all destroy some of the vitamins—in fact, the less you do to fruit, the more flavor and nourishment it will give you.

Freshly sliced mango, or peach, or strawberries in a glass bowl, topped with a dollop of whipped cream or frothy frozen yogurt make delicious desserts.

All the same, here are a few simple suggestions:

• If you like something sweet and cold to nibble on after a hot savory meal, cut a piece of watermelon into small squares and freeze.

• Cut a ripe, perfect banana into four or five pieces. Squeeze plenty of lemon juice onto each piece, wrap in individual squares of foil, and freeze.

• Put into the blender the following:
  1 glass orange juice
  1 apple, cut in pieces
  Juice of one lemon
  1 cup strawberries
  ½ cup yogurt

Blend until smooth. Pour into ice cube tray. When frozen, break into individual squares, put several into a pretty glass bowl, serve as dessert. (The whole recipe contains about 300 calories. Count the number of little squares to find out the calorie content of each.)

TABLE OF APPROXIMATE CALORIE CONTENT OF
3½ OUNCES OF FRUIT
(Fresh, raw, edible portions only)

	Calories
Apple	60
Apricot	55
Banana	90
Blackberry or blueberry	65
Cherry	80
Grapefruit	45
Grapes	75
Mango	75
Melon	35
Nectarine	70
Orange	55
Papaya	45
Peach	45
Pear	70
Pineapple	60
Plum	70
Raspberry	65
Strawberry	45
Tangerine	50
Watermelon	30

THE RESHAPE LUNCH RECIPES

These lunches are light, but far from skimpy! Our favorites have been variations of our "hot salad," served overflowing on a large dinner plate; or on cold winter days, a huge bowlful of thick creamy soup served with a crisp raw salad and a couple of crackers.

THE "HOT SALAD"

Wash and trim enough raw salad vegetables to line the bottom of a large dinner plate. (Shred the leafy greens, chop the other salad vegetables into bite-size pieces.) Spread 3 ounces of cottage cheese all over the vegetables, as if you were filling a pie.

Meanwhile, prepare your choice of cooked vegetables. In one cup of vegetable-extract broth,* steam half a pound of broccoli and mushrooms; or asparagus cut into 1-inch pieces; or any other nonstarchy vegetables singly or in combination. When just tender, drain well, straining the liquid into a cup. (Add chopped parsley and serve the broth as a first course.)

Spread the cooked vegetables over the cottage cheese. Sprinkle with lemon juice, herbs to taste, seasoned sea salt, and ½ tablespoon of oil.** Another delicious way of serving the "hot salad" is substituting either "Lecso," Ratatouille, or the Italian Mixed (see the Reshape Dinner Recipes) for the steamed vegetables. Either way, the blending of the cottage cheese and the hot, savory vegetables creates a satisfying, creamy consistency, while the raw, crunchy salad vegetables add an interesting texture. With the variety of ingredients, each mouthful is different, so that even though this is a huge dish, it is never boring.

THE CREAMY SOUPS

A recent study involving 500 dieters indicated that those whose diet included soup lost slightly more weight than those who did not eat soup. It seemed that the soup-eaters automatically consumed almost 100 calories a day *less* than the soupless dieters.

Why were the soup-eaters satisfied with less?

Soup is hot—it takes longer to eat, giving you longer eating pleasure. Soup is generous in volume—it fills you up. Soup leaves you with a cozy, warm feeling of satisfaction.

---

*In place of supermarket bouillon cubes, buy some high-protein vegetable extract at a health-food store. These come in powder form, they taste just like bouillon cubes, but they're probably better for your health.

**Instead of the oil, try half a teaspoon of mayonnaise blended into ¼ cup of plain yogurt. Or 1 tablespoon of catsup mixed into 2 tablespoons of sour cream. This is especially delicious over asparagus!

Each of our creamy soups adds up to about 160 calories. They're so rich, and they make such huge servings, that, served with a crisp salad and a couple of crackers, they're a meal in themselves. If half the quantity satisfies you, make up the difference by adding up to two ounces of chopped cooked chicken, or a crumbled hard-boiled egg.

Unless otherwise specified, for each of the creamy soups you will need half a pound of vegetables, 1½ cups water into which a bouillon cube* has been dissolved, 1½ teaspoons of butter, 1 teaspoon of flour, and 2 to 3 ounces of cottage cheese.

ASPARAGUS SOUP

Drop the asparagus (cut in 1-inch pieces) into 1½ cups of boiling water in which a bouillon cube or vegetable-extract powder has been dissolved. Simmer, uncovered, until asparagus is almost done. In a separate saucepan melt 1½ teaspoons butter, add 1 teaspoon flour, and 1 tablespoon chopped parsley. Stir constantly, diluting as needed with a little of the asparagus broth. When thoroughly blended, slowly add to the asparagus. Taste for salt. Simmer a few more minutes.

Reserving half the asparagus pieces, blend soup in blender with 2 to 3 ounces of cottage cheese (depending on the degree of creamy thickness you prefer). Return to saucepan with reserved asparagus pieces, heat through. Serve in huge bowl, or if you prefer, serve only one cupful poured over 2 ounces of cooked chicken or one chopped-up hard-boiled egg.

CAULIFLOWER SOUP

Separate the well-washed cauliflower into equal-sized flowerets, then proceed exactly the same as with the Asparagus Soup. Sprinkle with chopped parsley.

MUSHROOM SOUP

Sauté one small, finely chopped onion in the butter. Add the sliced mushrooms, and sauté until wilted. Slowly add the vegetable-extract broth, simmer gently. In a cup, mix the flour with a little of the mushroom liquid. When smoothly blended, stir into the soup. Simmer, partially covered, a few more minutes. Taste for salt.

Reserve half the mushroom slices. Put the rest of soup through blender, reheat, then top with the reserved mushroom slices. Instead of cottage cheese, serve with two tablespoons of sour cream.

Green Bean Soup

Bring the vegetable-extract broth to a boil. Drop in the green beans (cut in 1½-inch pieces), ½ clove of garlic, and ½ teaspoon lemon juice. Simmer until beans are nearly tender. Meanwhile, melt the butter, add ½ thinly sliced onion, sauté until translucent. Stir in flour and a little paprika and salt, stir for two or three minutes. Add a little of the bean broth, blend till smooth, then pour into the green beans and simmer another five minutes or so. Take soup from the stove, remove garlic, then proceed as for Asparagus and Cauliflower soups. Add more lemon, chopped dill to taste.

Savoy Cabbage Soup

Bring the vegetable-extract broth to a boil. Drop in the shredded savoy cabbage, simmer for ten minutes. Remove from heat. In separate saucepan, melt the butter, sprinkle with the flour, and proceed as for Asparagus and Cauliflower soups. Instead of the chicken pieces or the chopped egg, you may stir in an ounce of grated Swiss cheese, reheat and serve.

Tomato-Crème Soup

Scald and peel the tomatoes. (Make sure they're red, ripe tomatoes, but avoid overripe or bruised fruit.) Break them open and simmer in just a little of the vegetable-extract broth. When cooked, pass through a sieve. Melt the butter, sprinkle on the flour, stir for two or three minutes. Add the pureed tomatoes, stir in some more of the broth, cook, stirring for a few more minutes. Pour just a little of the soup into blender, blend with cottage cheese; return to saucepan, reheat, and serve over chopped hard-boiled egg. Sprinkle with chopped parsley.

Spring-Vegetable Soup

Use a mixture of green peas, carrots, and a small potato, to a total of ½ pound in weight. In separate saucepan, simmer ¼ pound of cauliflower in one cup of the vegetable-extract broth, while the chopped carrot, peas, and chopped potato are simmering in another ¾ cup. In a small saucepan melt the butter, sprinkle on the flour, a dash of paprika, and stir for two or three minutes. Slowly add to cooked cauliflower, pour into blender. Blend until smooth. Reheat together with the mixed chopped vegetables. Just before serving, blend a table-spoonful of sour cream with a little of the soup, return to saucepan, and serve.

Whether you serve yourself the whole huge bowlful of soup only, or half the quantity of soup with meat or egg, a small dish of crisp lettuce, cucumber, and celery will complement the richness of the soup and complete the meal with practically no additional calories.

For a complete change of pace, here's a delicious Hungarian fish soup that's very low in calories.

Halaszle ("Fisherman's Soup")
Your portion: 200 calories

1 fresh carp, boned; flesh cut into chunks
1 medium onion, thinly sliced
Dash of paprika
A little sour cream
1 green pepper, medium size
1 small hot pepper
1 large tomato

Weigh the chunks of fish. Count how many pieces make four ounces: This is what you will eat. (Reserve the rest *after* they've cooked in the soup.) Put all the pieces of fish in a large bowl, sprinkle with salt, and set aside.

Put onion slices in a medium-size saucepan, cover with fish head and bones, pour on enough water to cover. Add paprika and bring to a simmer. After half an hour, strain into the pot with the fish chunks. Add sliced peppers, peeled and chopped tomato. Keep simmering, *without stirring,* but shaking gently from side to side now and then. When fish flakes easily, remove from heat and let stand for ten minutes. Serve with a little sour cream.

Here's a Hot Tip to Help You Lose Weight Fast

Once a week during Stage One, or whenever you want to speed up the weight-loss process, make up a big potful of our extrarich Super Soup and eat nothing else all day. The recipe that follows makes five to six cups of soup, at a total of 280 calories for the whole day!

Super Soup

3 cups of water
1 tablespoon caraway seeds
1 teaspoon vegetable protein powder
1½ pounds cauliflower
1 medium tomato
3 tablespoons minced parsley
1 clove garlic
6 ounces cottage cheese

Add caraway seeds and protein powder to the water, bring to the boil. Thinly slice the cauliflower, quarter the tomato. Add vegetables and garlic to the water, simmer until cauliflower is just tender (about five minutes). Reserve some of the cooked cauliflower. Put the rest of the soup into the blender, add the cottage cheese, and blend until very smooth. Return to the reserved cauliflower, sprinkle with a little more chopped parsley.

Whenever you feel hungry, heat a small bowlful of the Super Soup, sprinkle with fresh parsley, enjoy. (Sip it from a teaspoon, you'll enjoy even more its delicious flavor and rich texture.)

THE RESHAPE DINNER RECIPES

Green Beans Fözelék

1 pound green beans
1 teaspoon vegetable extract powder
1 teaspoon flour
1 medium tomato, cut in halves
1 clove garlic, minced
2 tablespoons finely minced dill
Lemon juice to taste
2 tablespoons sour cream

Cut the cleaned and trimmed green beans into 1-inch pieces. In 1¼ cup of water, dissolve the vegetable extract, bring broth to boil. Add beans, tomato halves, and minced garlic, reduce heat and simmer until beans are quite tender. (If needed, add more water.) Discard tomato. Remove a few spoonfuls of the sauce into a cup and stir in flour. Blend it until smooth, then very gradually add to the beans, stir. Simmer until sauce has thickened. Add dill and lemon juice, check seasoning. Remove from heat, carefully blend in sour cream.

Spinach Gemüse

1 pound spinach, cleaned (must be young, tender)
1 clove garlic, bruised
2 heaping teaspoons butter
1 teaspoon flour
½ cup milk plus a little of the spinach water, as needed
Pinch of nutmeg

Steam the cleaned spinach in the water that's left clinging to the leaves after washing, together with the garlic. When spinach is quite limp, discard the garlic and drain the spinach, reserving the liquid. Press out every last drop of liquid. Coarsely chop the spinach. Melt the butter over low heat, stir in flour, and cook, then gradually add the milk, the nutmeg, and ¼ cup of spinach water; simmer for about ten minutes, frequently stirring. Add the spinach, stir thoroughly, adjust seasoning, and serve. If you can afford the extra calories, just before serving add half of a well-beaten egg while stirring continuously.

Green Peas Fözelék

Taste the peas before you buy them, to make sure they're young and sweet. Buy about two pounds in the pod—if that's too much, you can always use the surplus in another dish.

½ pound shelled peas
1 tablespoon butter
Finely chopped parsley
1 level teaspoon flour
Salt

Rinse the peas under cold water. Drop them into 1 cup boiling water, bring back to simmer and cook, uncovered, until tender. Drain, but reserve the liquid. Gently melt the butter, stir in parsley and flour. Cook for a couple of minutes, then slowly add the cooking liquid and simmer for ten minutes. Add the cooked peas, remove from heat, and serve.

Squash Fözelék

1 pound zucchini or yellow summer squash
Few slices onion
1 tablespoon oil
1 teaspoon flour
½ teaspoon paprika
1 tablespoon chopped fresh dill
Lemon juice to taste
1 tablespoon sour cream

Cut the peeled zucchini or squash into long, thin strips, sprinkle with salt, and set aside for twenty minutes in a glass or porcelain bowl. In medium saucepan, sauté the onion in the oil, press liquid from squash and add; simmer until squash wilts. Sprinkle with the flour and paprika and keep turning for two or three minutes over low heat. Gradually add one cup of warm water and continue to simmer, uncovered, for five minutes. Add the chopped dill and lemon juice to taste. Remove from heat and allow to cool. Very carefully blend in the sour cream, adjust seasoning, and serve.

Carrot Fözelék

¾ pound carrots
2 heaping teaspoons butter
1 teaspoon flour
½ cup skim milk
½ teaspoon honey (optional)

Wash and scrape the carrots, grate them coarsely or cut them into very thin slices. Melt the butter and, adding a little water, sauté carrots, covered, until quite soft. Sprinkle with the flour and continue to sauté. Slowly add the milk, bring to the boil, simmer for a few minutes, and serve. Add salt only at the table to prevent milk from curdling. Sweeten with the honey if you wish.

CAULIFLOWER GEMÜSE

¾ pound cauliflower
1 tablespoon butter
1 teaspoon flour
Chopped parsley
½ cup skim milk
1 tablespoon sour cream

Wash cauliflower, break into uniform-size flowerets. Drop them into salted, boiling water, cook rapidly, uncovered, for about fifteen minutes. Strain, reserving broth. Rinse in cold water, drain. Melt butter in medium saucepan over low heat. Add the parsley and flour, cook for few minutes. Gradually stir in ½ cup of the cauliflower broth and the milk and continue cooking over low heat, stirring often. When sauce has thickened, add drained cauliflower and remove from heat. Very carefully blend in sour cream and serve.

GREEN PEPPER AND TOMATO "LECSO" (LEH-CHO)

½ pound green pepper strips
½ pound peeled, cored, and quartered tomatoes
1 small onion, finely chopped
1 tablespoon oil
2 frankfurters, cut in rings
1 teaspoon paprika, a little salt

Sauté the finely chopped onion in the oil until onion starts to wilt. Sprinkle on the paprika and salt and cook a little longer. Stir in the vegetables, cover, and simmer until green pepper is tender, about twenty minutes. Stir in the frankfurter rings and simmer ten minutes more. (Counts as meat dish)

Ratatouille

1 pound of vegetables made up of medium onion, zucchini,
 eggplant, green pepper, and tomatoes
1 clove garlic, chopped
1½ tablespoons oil (preferably olive oil)
Chopped parsley
Basil (fresh or dried)

Cook sliced onion and chopped garlic in the oil. Add sliced
zucchini, cubed eggplant, chopped green pepper, and peeled
and diced tomatoes. Sprinkle with salt, parsley, and basil, cover
and simmer fifteen minutes. Uncover and cook until vegetables
are tender and juice is thickened.

Italian Mixed Vegetables

1 pound of vegetables made up of tomatoes, carrot,
 zucchini, corn from the cob, green pepper, a few slices
 onions, a small potato
1 tablespoon oil
1 teaspoon oregano leaves
1 teaspoon flour

Scald, peel, and chop the tomatoes, thinly slice the carrot and
zucchini, dice the potato, cut the green pepper into strips. Place
all the ingredients into a saucepan, cover and simmer for fifteen
to twenty minutes, until potatoes are tender. Remove a little of
the liquid, cool, blend in the flour. Return to saucepan, simmer
a little while longer.

Here's a trick worth remembering:

Any recipe, including the Reshape Recipes, which begins
with ". . . sauté in 1 tablespoon (or more) of oil," may be made
even more calorie-sparing by substituting two tablespoons of
vegetable-extract broth for the oil at the beginning of the recipe.
Continue as directed, then add just one teaspoon of oil at the

end, when you've taken the dish from the heat. The flavor is almost as rich, and you've saved yourself some sixty to eighty calories. Use this method when you're adding "Lecso," Ratatouille, or the Italian Mixed to your "hot salad." The creaminess of the cottage cheese will make up for the slight lack of richness.

What To Do When You're Eating Out

On days when you're eating out at night, skip breakfast but have your usual 200-calorie lunch. This means that you'll have 600 calories up your sleeve to spend on your dinner.

At the restaurant, order soup—the richest soup on the menu. Make sure it is a protein soup such as lentil, bean, minestrone, or cream of chicken with plenty of chicken pieces floating in it. Such a soup will have up to 300 calories, but it will stop you from feeling deprived since its volume will fill your stomach, and its high calorie count will inform your satiety control center that you have already eaten and are quite satisfied. It takes about twenty-five minutes for this information to reach your brain, so by the time the next course comes around, you won't feel hungry any more. The remaining 300 calories will be enough to cover a discreet nibble at whatever is next on your plate, as you quite truthfully explain to your dinner partners: "That soup was so rich and filling, I'm just not hungry any more."

Use the same delayed-satiety syndrome when you're invited and cannot choose your menu. Simply eat the protein-richest food to begin with, then just play with the rest of your plate till hunger disappears.

Some Important Pointers to Help You to Lost Weight Quickly and Steadily

1. Don't try to cut down on your salad and vegetable dishes in order to save calories. If you do, you'll wind up feeling un-

satisfied, and you'll suddenly find yourself eating other things much higher in calories. Remember, there is simply no other category of food that is as calorie sparing relative to bulk as nature's vitamin and mineral powerhouse: the vegetable! Don't stretch your stomach, but do eat enough of your vegetable dishes to feel fully satisfied.

2. When you've finished your meal, get up from the table and *immediately* march into the bathroom to brush your teeth and rinse your mouth. Don't clean up first, don't even approach the kitchen (some of us, no matter how well filled we feel, just cannot bring ourselves to throw anything out, and it's easier to swallow a few mouthfuls of leftovers than to store them in the refrigerator!) but go straight to the bathroom (or the washroom at work). The more you fuss with your teeth, the less likely you'll be to spoil the effect by snacking. Floss carefully, massage the gums, rinse with a pleasant-tasting mouthwash. The clean fresh taste in your mouth will keep you from snacking until the next meal.

3. On rare days when you just cannot keep to your low calorie allowance for whatever reason, be sure not to go over your no-gain–no-loss "maintenance" allowance. At this stage, this is simply your basic daily calorie requirement as calculated by multiplying your "ideal weight" by 12 if you're under fifty years old, or by 11 if you're over. (In Stage Two of the Reshape Program we will establish your fixed "maintenance" allowance with much greater precision.) In this way, if you make little progress on that day—and as long as you perform your other Reshape activities faithfully, you'll still be making some progress—at least you won't be going backward.

4. Should you ever go on a real binge, compensate with a semifast the following day by eating nothing but firm, ripe tomatoes sprinkled with your favorite herb. (No more than 1½ pounds of tomatos for the whole day.) Just before you go to bed, sip a glass of warm skim milk into which you've stirred a teaspoonful of blackstrap molasses. This will give you some protein and other nutrients, and calcium to promote peaceful sleep.

If you prefer, you may semifast on three small glasses of orange juice instead of the tomatoes, or on any other raw fruit or vegetable, as long as your total calorie intake for the day, not counting the warm milk with molasses, is no more than 150 calories. (The milk drink will add another 100 calories. Do have it though, for undisturbed sleep is important for the success of any undertaking—and that goes for the Reshape Program too!) Or if you like, gorge yourself on nothing but Super Soup all day.

5. If you wish to accelerate your weight reduction, go on one of the semifasts as described above one day a week, then enjoy your big, rich Reshape Meals all the rest of the week.

6. Remember, if you're losing too much weight on an 800-calorie diet, or if your height allows you more calories, make up the difference in *protein* foods (meat, fish, poultry, or cheese) and *fruit*—not in bread, cereals, cookies, and the like.

A Chastity Belt for the Mouth?

The knight of old, when he rode off into battle, clamped an iron belt on his beloved to keep her chaste from the waist down should a handsome rake come a-courting during his absence.

We ladies of the twentieth century are more concerned with resisting temptation from the neck up. According to reports, some women have actually had their jaws wired shut to keep themselves from eating! We have found that an imaginary mouth-clamp can do wonders for compulsive snackers.

Here's what you do.

As soon as you've finished a meal, imagine that a tight clamp with a lock is fitted to your gullet. The key that fastens the lock is the act of brushing your teeth. Once the clamp is safely locked— once you've brushed your teeth—no food can pass down your throat until the clamp is unlocked again. How do you unlock it? By inserting one small green olive into your mouth.

Keep the key to the lock—the single olive—out of easy reach, and only pop it into your mouth in order to unlock the phantom chastity belt when your next meal is due. (It also serves as a tasty little appetizer!) You can condition yourself to such an extent that you won't feel like eating at all unless stimulated by the one green olive!

Here's another tip: Should you ever feel hungry while the "belt" is "locked," place your index fingers into your ears, palms facing forward, so that the balls of your fingers rest against the little bits of cartilage that project from your ears. Now close in with your thumbs, and firmly massage these projections between index finger and thumb until hunger stops (one or two minutes). This little trick will stop you from breaking the lock on your imaginary chastity belt. (So when your knight returns, you may not be so chaste, but you'll be *slim!*)

10

Things to Do Throughout the Day

Bottoms Up!

Toast yourself with a glass of water several times during the morning—whenever you feel you'd like something to eat! Use spring water or filtered water, as in most localities ordinary tap water contains too many chemicals. Do not drink water immediately before a meal—fifteen minutes in between is about right—and do not drink with meals, nor for about two hours after, as water dilutes the digestive juices in the stomach and therefore interferes with optimum digestion. Never gulp the water, but sip it slowly. If you like, you can squeeze some lemon into your drink for refreshing flavor. Whenever you can do so, drink in a horizontal position, with your legs elevated, and stay in that position for ten to fifteen minutes.

Relax

While you're in the horizontal position, take some deep breaths—*in* slowly through the nose, *out* sharply through the mouth; continue deep-breathing slowly and rhythmically, and relaxing, one by one, all the muscles in your face and body. Remember to get up gradually and sit for a minute before you get to your feet.

Practice the Reshape Posture

Remind yourself as often as you can to practice the Reshape Posture. Head straight, shoulders dropped, stomach in, tail tucked under. Breathing deeply and rhythmically, point to an imaginary spot a little above and out from the tips of your breasts, then pretend you're trying to touch your breasts to your pointing fingers. Use chest muscles only. Do this when you're standing, sitting, or even lying down. Practice the posture without actually pointing your fingers (just imagine you are pointing). If you breathe deeply while you practice the Reshape Posture, you'll learn to keep your muscles *relaxed* in the proper position. This is important—we don't want a tense body leading to fatigue and other potential problems.

Massage When No One's Looking

Rolls of fat on tummy, on hips, on tops of thighs, and "love handles" around the midriff can do with some additional surreptitious massaging any old time during the day. As you work, or read, or watch television, knead them, pinch them between fingers and thumb, then stroke in the direction of the heart. But take care not to bruise.

While the Kettle Boils

Make it a habit to always *use* waiting time. In the kitchen, while you're waiting for your breakfast egg to boil, or for your vegetables to cook, hold on to the counter and do vigorous leg-lifts, ten to each side. If you happen to have a radio in your kitchen, do a few minutes of disco-dancing, making sure to shiver and shake, stretch and bump in all directions.

The Goose Step and the Duck Walk

Moving in your house from room to room, don't just walk, goose-step. Lift your forward leg as high as you can, pointing your toes and keeping your knees straight. Or bend your knees until you're in a half-squatting position, and walk in this modified duck-walk stance.

At Work, Waiting at a Stop Light, Watching Television

Stretch your arms horizontally, palms facing forward, and push against an imaginary wall. Keep pushing as you move your arms gradually to the sides, then above your head, then even behind you as far as you can, keeping that imaginary wall from closing around you.

To firm insides of thighs, place your fists between your knees and try to squeeze them together, pressing with your thigh muscles as hard as you can.

To massage inside of knees, slap them together.

In the next few weeks you'll see tremendous changes in your body. Weight and inches will be slipping away from you at a steady rate. You'll see rolls of fat disappearing from your "bulge" areas, and you'll notice a fantastic difference in the tone and feel of your body.

You'll enjoy Stage One of your figure Reshape; I know *we* did. The laziest of us thirty-seven pretty-lazy ladies couldn't wait to get on with all the routines, with the great meals, with the exercises—and with the daily weigh-in and measure-up ritual. What could be more electrifying than watching your figure getting closer and closer to the fabulous new *you!*

So go to it. Follow the easy Stage One Summary until weight and inches are down . . . down where you want them!

See you in Stage Two.

Summary—

STAGE ONE

What You'll Need:

Broom
Four pillows or one pillow and three folded blankets
Bathroom scale
Tape measure
3 plastic kitchen bags, size 2' x 2'6"
Cord to tie around waist
Pair of stretch briefs
Pair of old pantyhose or ballet tights
Pair of warm-up pants
Exercise book and pen

For your meals:
Variety of herbs
Vegetable-protein seasoning

A hearty appetite and a will to create a fabulous body!

In-Bed Exercises
Total time: 5 minutes
(Details on page 64)

1. *The S-T-R-E-T-C-H:* yawn; bend, rotate feet.
   Clasp hands behind neck. Without pausing, do up to ten each:
2. *The Vertical Leg-Lift:* legs together, straight, toes pointing
3. *The Knees-to-Chest:* legs together, toes pointing
4. *The Scissors:* alternate legs, knees straight, raise, lower.
   Rest briefly
5. *The Isometric Ankle-Cross:* hold to a count of six, reverse
6. *The Isometric Wrist Push and Wrist Pull:* ten times each, hold each to a count of six.

123

Stretching–Firming
Total time: 3 minutes
(Details on page 71)

Open the window. Grab a broom.
1. *The Reach for the Ceiling*
2. *The Side Twist:* ten double bumps, ten single bumps in each direction
3. *The Side Bend:* ten doubles, ten singles, in each direction
4. *The Backward and Forward Bend:* ten doubles, ten singles, in each direction
* *First Hard Call for Energy: 25 Jumps* (clap palms together above your head, spread feet)

Hand Massage
Total time: 20 minutes
(Details on page 77)

Relax on pillows, hips elevated, legs highest
1. *Finger Pressure*
    • rotate foot
    • rotate each toe
    • rub with thumb above toe-line
    • massage whole foot
    • press around heel and ankle
2. *Massage of Thighs, Hips, Buttocks*
   Start with the heavier leg. Be careful not to bruise. Always stroke in the direction of the heart. Alternate:
    • Gentle stroking
    • Kneading
    • Scoring
    • Slapping
   *Second Hard Call for Energy: 10 Knee-Bends

Floor Massage
Total time: 3 minutes
(Details on page 79)

At least twenty-five of each:
1. *The Side Roll:* knees together, legs bent, hands behind you
2. *The Side Rock:* knees apart, feet close to body, hands on ankles
3. *The Fanny Press:* knees together, legs bent, hands behind you. Finish with ten bicycle kicks, then rest, hips elevated, legs highest.

Friction Massage and Putting On
the Slimming Pants
Total time: 8 minutes
(Details on page 84)

1. *Hip-Bath:* in comfortably hot water, massage hips, thighs, and buttocks with loofah or rough washcloth
2. *Pat Dry*
3. *Slimming Pants*
   a. Slip on first plastic bag
   b. Tie at waist with cord
   c. Slip stretch briefs over plastic bag
   d. Slip on two remaining plastic bags, one on each leg
   e. Tuck tops of bags into stretch briefs
   f. Pull firm pantyhose over all, to hold in place
   e. Pull on fleecy warm-up pants

Things To Do While Your Slimming
Pants Are Working
Total time: 15 minutes
(Details on page 86)

1. *Run, Skip, Jump* for up to ten minutes (Third Extra-Hard Call for Energy)
   Rest, horizontal
2. *Antigravity Position*
   Rest, horizontal
3. *Wall Massage:* bump "riding breeches" up to a hundred times on each side
4. *Broom-Handle Massage*
5. *Slap* all over massaged areas
6. *Bicycle* in the air
7. Rest, hips elevated, legs highest

Diet
(Details on page 96)

Drink bottled or filtered water, 4 to 6 glasses throughout the day.

Write Here Your Daily Calorie Allowance (as worked
out according to rules on page 31) ....
Less 500 calories for quick weight-loss ....500 _____

YOUR DAILY STAGE ONE QUOTA: _____

The basic 800-calories-a-day meal structure:

BREAKFAST	1 egg or equivalent	70
(pages 97-98)	1 slice whole wheat bread	55
	1 serving of fruit	50
		Total: 175

LUNCH	Cooked vegetables	50
(pages 105-110)	3 ounces ½ percent butterfat cottage cheese	60
	Oil or butter, ½ tablespoon	60
	Cracker	30
		Total: 200

DINNER	3 ounces poultry or fish	120
(pages 111-115)	Creamy vegetable *Gemüse*	255
	Fruit dessert	50
		Total: 425

IMPORTANT:	If your quota allows *more,* increase protein & fruit. If your quota allows *less,* keep proportions, eat less

After a Meal, Immediately Brush Your Teeth!

Some Things To Do Throughout The Day:
(Details on Page 120)

1. Practice Reshape Posture
2. Massage rolls of fat on tummy, hips, thighs
3. Relax, breathing deeply
4. Slap knees together
5. Squeeze fists between knees
6. Drink water
7. If you're hungry, drink clear, hot vegetable broth
8. Stretch . . . s-t-r-e-t-c-h
9. Do some disco-dancing
10. Think about your terrific new wardrobe and all the things you'll do once you have your fabulous figure!

11

If Your Weight Is Right But Your Basic Shape Is Still Wrong . . .

Before we go on to Stage Two of the Reshape Program, let's stop for a moment and consider: What if you've reached your ideal weight, but your hips or thighs are still outside your ideal measurements?

First, you must rule out the possibility that the width of your pelvis will preclude any further slimming in the hip area.

Feel the hipbones with your fingers. Can you feel the bone? Is there still considerable padding between bone and skin, or are you rolling nothing but a thin layer of tissue between your fingers?

If the hipbone and the bones where the thighs meet the trunk have only thin layers of skin, then obviously in those areas you have reached your limits. That does not mean, however, that you can't still slim the buttocks and the thighs.

Have a good look at your face. Unless your rapid weight-loss has caused your face to become too thin, which is unlikely, you can safely go two to three pounds *under* your ideal weight. Simply follow the Reshape routine for a few more days, and if the last inches are too stubborn, go on a semifast (tomatoes only several times a day, and warm skim milk with blackstrap molasses before bed at night) one day in the week. Before long, the last stubborn inches, too, will disappear.

If you feel that you've lost too much weight too rapidly, then go on to Stage Two and stabilize your weight at its present stage for a few weeks. Then before going on to Stage Three, go back to Stage One for a few days. If you like, you can repeat this procedure a few times, until the last few inches are lost. Remember, the more your cells learn to give up their fat content in a particular area, the more readily they will do so. In the past, whenever I had managed to lose quite a bit of weight, through rigorous dieting and conventional exercising, it came off all other parts of my body but my hip-thigh-buttocks area. Since I Reshaped my figure, I never put on more than two to three pounds, and when I take them off in just a few days, my bottom and thighs are the first to slim!

So stop and go as often as you like, but be sure to carry out all the Reshape activities as directed, with particular attention to your problem areas during the slimming stage. If you've been using your slimming pants once a week only during the later part of your Stage One period, now use them every day again for a while. Semifast occasionally if you like. Raise your running-jumping-skipping routine to twelve or fifteen minutes, with a few minutes of rest (in the horizontal position, with legs raised) at half time. Rest in the antigravity position several times during the day, especially after exercise, and in the periods two to four hours after a meal, when the nutrients have entered the bloodstream and fat deposition is most likely to occur.

Needless to say, keep your food pure and simple and continue drinking three to four large glasses of pure water (or water with lemon juice), if possible in the horizontal position, with your legs raised. Observe the Reshape *timing* and the Reshape *sequence* of the activities as directed, and you'll find that the last stubborn inches on hips, thighs, and buttocks will disappear, even if you haven't lost more (and you shouldn't!) than two to three extra pounds under your ideal weight.

PART III

The Woman's Total Reshape Program—

STAGE TWO

STABILIZE NEW LOW WEIGHT FOR
ALWAYS; CORRECT
LONG-STANDING POSTURE
FAULTS; BUILD UP SELECTED
MUSCLES FOR SUPER SHAPE AND
AS FOUNDATION FOR FUTURE
BUSTLINE

12

Let's Take a Good Look at Posture

Now that we've carved away the disfiguring fat, we can take a good look at your basic body line and see what needs to be done to make it really terrific.

The basic framework of the body is, of course, the skeleton. The skeleton gives the body shape, it protects the organs, and it provides the movable parts that make it possible for you to sit, stand, walk, and so forth. Attached to the skeleton and causing the bones to move are the skeletal muscles. It is the size, shape, and condition of these skeletal muscles that determine *how* attractively you sit, stand, walk, and so on. Muscles that become stretched or weak allow your skeleton to slump and your organs to spill out of their proper positions; muscles that become shortened and tense create unattractive body lines as well as fatigue and possibly even ill health. Fortunately, muscle, unlike the bony skeleton itself, lends itself marvelously to deliberate, systematic improvement: Stretched muscles can be made to shorten and gain strength; short, tense muscles can be stretched; and weak, insignificant muscles can be built up to many times their original size. At this stage of our body-shaping process, we will work on the muscles with two distinct purposes in mind: to eradicate long-standing posture faults, and to build attractive shape into calves, thighs, chest, and arms, as needed.

133

Take a Critical Look at Your Posture

For a really fabulous figure, you must carry yourself superbly! No doubt losing the rolls of fat on tummy and buttocks, and practicing the Reshape Posture, have already done a lot for your carriage. But if you have long-standing posture-problems, this is the time to work on them.

Standing in front of a full-length mirror with your clothes off and in your bare feet, turn sideways to the mirror and compare your posture to the illustrations. Observe the position of the head, the neck, and the shoulders—is *your* head slumped forward? Or too far back, with chin pointing too high? Compare.

Is your back naturally straight, or is it curved, the shoulders sagging? Is your tummy as flat as it should be? Or does it sag forward, protruding at the middle? What about your buttocks? Neatly tucked under, or sticking out?

Turn to face the mirror. Are your legs straight or are you knock-kneed? Ankles turning in or out? Toes pointing outward or inward?

The following are common posture problems. Identify your own; then note the special exercises designed to correct them.

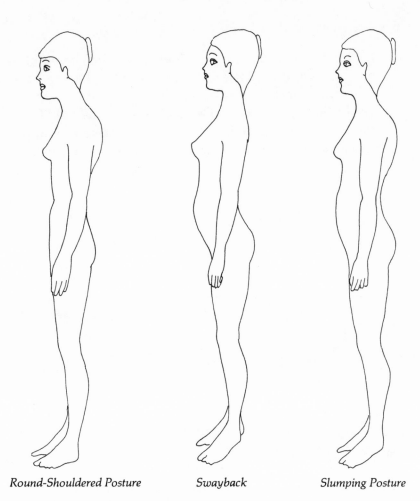

Round-Shouldered Posture   *Swayback*   *Slumping Posture*

1. Round-Shouldered Posture
   This posture affects the upper part of the back, which is
   rounded; the shoulders, which fall forward; and the neck,
   which tends to protrude, causing the head to tilt backward
   and the chin to push forward and up.

   Remedy for round-shouldered posture:
   a. Place a small cushion on the floor. Lie on your back, in
      such a way that the cushion is under your shoulder blades
      and the back and top of your head touches the floor. Relax
      your neck and shoulder muscles, let them go completely.
      Stay in this position for three minutes.

b. Lie on the floor, face down. Hold your hands behind the back of your head. Raise your elbows off the floor and pull them back as far as you can without discomfort. Now raise your head and chest as far back as you can and hold for as long as you're able. Relax. Breathe in . . . raise your upper trunk again as far as you can . . . breathe out and relax.

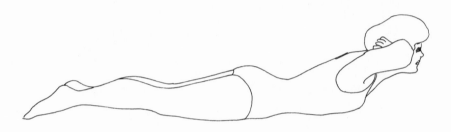

REMEMBER: Do not stretch further than you can without discomfort. When you've reached your comfortable limit, stop, relax, then *repeat*. With each repetition, you'll reach further and further, until you can do your maximum with ease.

2. Slumping Posture

In this posture not only are the shoulders and upper back rounded, and the head tilted back, but the pelvis is tilted forward, the abdomen protrudes, and the buttocks stick out at the back.

Remedy for slumping posture:

a. Since this posture includes a rounded upper back and shoulders, the previous two exercises (for round-shouldered posture) apply equally well. For the pelvic area, do the following:

b. Get down on your hands and knees. Drop your head down between your arms, and at the same time arch your *lower* back like a cat. Then let your pelvic area sink *downward* while you bring your head and neck *up*. Repeat in such a way that the repetitions form a rhythmic rocking. Arch . . . relax . . . arch . . . relax.

c. In the same position, rock your pelvis sideways, right, left, right, left, without lifting or even moving your thighs.

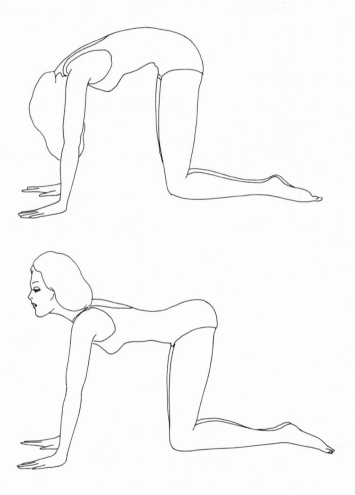

d. Stand up. Bend forward, let your head and arms hang loosely toward the floor. Now very slowly uncurl your spine, beginning at the base, until you're erect. Look at your profile in the mirror. Hold the position. Repeat whenever you can think of it, and try to maintain the position indefinitely.

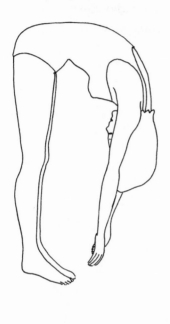

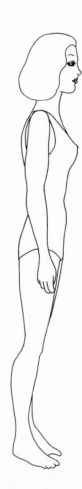

3. Swayback

As in the slumping posture, the swayback also demonstrates a protruding tummy and behind, though the upper back and shoulder positions may be quite acceptable.

Remedy for the swayback:

a. Lie on your back, knees bent, soles of your feet flat on the floor, arms relaxed by your side. Press your lower back hard against the floor, hold, relax . . . hold . . . relax. Repeat several times.

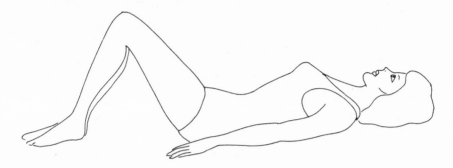

b. From a standing position, drop your head and arms toward the floor. Inhale, and as you do so, contract your abdomen. Exhale and relax. Inhale . . . contract; exhale . . . relax. As you're doing this, you will feel a sensation of expansion and contraction in your lower back. To come up, uncurl slowly, one vertebra at a time, and when erect, hold the position. Do this latter exercise several times a day, until the posture becomes permanent.

4. Knock-knees and/or Flat Feet
   All kind of foot problems benefit from walking barefooted on a soft carpet or, better still, in the sand on the beach. Try to walk on the water's edge, where the damp sand has some "give."

   Remedy for knock-knees and flat feet:
   Walk on the outer edges of your feet.

5. Bowlegs and Outward Curving Ankles
   Remedy: Walk (on carpet or on the beach) with your weight on the inside of your feet.

6. Turned-in Toes or Turned-out Toes
   Whichever your problem, practice walking around the room
   with your toes pointing the opposite way (*inward* if you tend
   to stand like a duck, *outward* if you're pigeon-toed).

Now that you've identified your posture problems and their
remedies, go to page 161 in the Summary and mark the posture
exercises you will be incorporating into your daily Reshape
routine. Check your posture several times during the day in a
full-length mirror, both full-face and in profile. If your shoulders
are held too high, rotate them a few times in their sockets first
forward, then backward, then let them drop, relaxed. If your
neck seems tense and stiff, drop your head limply forward,
chin-to-chest . . . then bring your head up straight slowly.
Repeat. Rotate your arms, then your hands from the wrists, then
your feet, then drop each limb gently, in a perfectly relaxed
state. Learn to relax each part of your body whether you're lying
down, or sitting, or even standing up. Drop your head and arms
forward toward the floor, bending from the waist; swing
loosely, then uncurl very slowly until you're erect but relaxed.
Then assume the Reshape Posture as you were doing it in Stage
One.

13

You Don't Want to Be a Ms. Universe, But...

Now that your weight is what you want it to be, you may find that your thighs or calves are actually thinner than the chart prescribes. This may be cause for rejoicing; however, have a good look at your body. Thin is not always beautiful. You may need some shapely muscle to give your limbs exciting contours!

Hormones prevent women developing the kind of rippling, bulging muscles male weight lifters are so proud of. Also, it is claimed that women's skin is thicker than men's, so that enlarged muscles show through as attractive curves. In the previous chapter you had a good long look at your new thin body and pinpointed whatever posture faults you may have. This time, concentrate on the lack of shape, if any, of your thighs and calves, your arms, and the upper part of your chest. Which parts need building up? Note the remedying exercises and mark them on page 162 in the Summary.

How Muscles Are Made to Grow

Body builders explain that contrary to what many people think, muscles do not grow while they're being exercised. During exercise, the muscle tissues are broken down and carried away in the bloodstream. During the next twenty-four hours or so, the broken-down tissues will be replaced—and since your body has taken note of the new increased demand made on that muscle, the replacement will be stronger and thicker than the tissue it replaces. This explains why body builders work a particular area one day and allow it to rest on the next day—it is during the period of rest that the tissue is being replaced—and also why the demand on the muscle has to be gradually increased. With each increase in demand, extra bulk is added; the gradual increase in demand is easiest effected by the addition of weights to barbells or dumbbells.

If you happen to have access to a set of weights (husband's, son's, or lover's), then of course you should use them. If not, here's a simple set you can put together with parts you probably have at home.

Your Homemade Set of Weights

Take two empty half-gallon plastic bottles, the kind you buy milk or juice in. Put them on your kitchen scales, one at a time, and add water until each registers two pounds. Screw the cap on very tightly and use as dumbbells. They're slender enough to grip in your hands; or you can hold them by their grips. For a barbell, simply hang the bottles on the two ends of your broomstick, making sure that they're exactly at the same distance from the ends, and taping them there. The broomstick fits snugly through the grips of the bottles, helping them to stay in place. With this system, you simply add water as you need to increase from two pounds to three, then to four. Since they each hold over four pounds, you won't need to go on to anything heavier. (You could, of course, use the one-gallon bottles, which weigh about ten pounds each when full with water, but you must not lift weights more than about five pounds without expert supervision. Nor is it necessary for our purposes.)

For your ankle-weights, simply fill two long, narrow plastic bags (of the kind you get your newspaper delivered in) with beans, or lentils, or some other grain-type, heavy substance, until they weigh exactly two pounds each. Lay them on a table. Press out all the air, then close them with twist-ties about two inches from the ends. Now pick up the other ends and letting the contents run toward the center, tie twist-ties about two inches from these ends, too. You'll have something like two sausages, with ties at two inches from both ends. Now you can simply drape them around your ankles, and secure the two ends with more twist-ties. (For extra strength, use double plastic bags, one inside the other.)

How Much Weight Should You Use?

Body builders, who aim mainly for superior strength, use very heavy weights, and not too many repetitions in each "set." But for size and shape, ten repetitions repeated three times with a minute's rest between the "sets" is the approach favored by many experts, with the weight used depending on the individual's strength. The important thing is that you should be able to do the ten repetitions without involving other muscles, but at the same time the last two or three repetitions must be something of an effort. If they're not, then a little more weight should be added. (An extra cup of water in your plastic bottles!) Since you're already in pretty good shape from your previous Reshape activities, you can start with two pounds and work up to four or five pounds per bottle.

Pick out the areas you need to add extra shape to, then make a note of the exercises and mark them in the Summary. (You're almost certain to benefit from the exercises that develop the chest. They build muscles, expand the rib cage, increase lung capacity, and in general provide a magnificent foundation for your new bustline. So be sure to include them in your weight-lifting routine.)

1. THE UPPER ARMS

The Curl. Stand up straight, feet slightly apart, barbell held in both hands at thigh-level, your palms pointing forward. Now bend your elbows, thereby *curling* the barbell to shoulder height. Be sure all the work is done by the muscles of the upper arms. Repeat ten times. Rest for one minute. Perform two more "sets" of ten repetitions each.

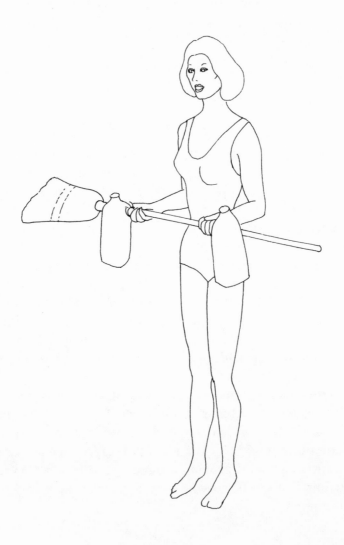

2. THE CHEST
   a. Bench Press. Place a blanket on a coffee table. Lie on your
      back in such a way that your feet are solidly on the ground.
      Lift the barbell at arm's length over your chest and
      hold—this is your starting position. Now inhale and lower
      the barbell to your chest as you do so. Exhale as you press
      the barbell up to the starting position. (NOTE: Watch that
      you hold the barbell over your *chest*, not over your eyes.
      Also, keep your body flat on the table, without raising
      buttocks or arching off it. If you're unable to do so, take
      some of the water out of the bottles, being cautious to keep
      them at equal weight.) Repeat ten times. Lower the barbell
      to your thighs and rest. Do two more sets of ten.

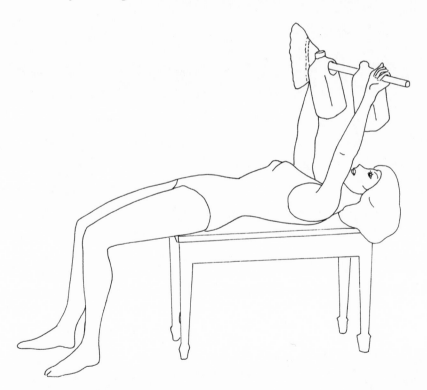

b. Pullover with Dumbbells. Lying on the coffee table with the top of your head just over the end and the soles of your feet firmly on the ground (if your coffee table is too long, lie *across*, with only your back resting on the table; keep your hips low, as the illustration shows), grab the two bottles firmly and hold them, with your arms bent, by your sides just below the bust. Inhaling deeply, filling your chest as high as you can, raise the "dumbbells" up and back, until they're behind your head, almost touching the floor. Keeping your chest high, exhale as you return to starting position. Do ten repetitions, rest. Continue until you've completed three sets.

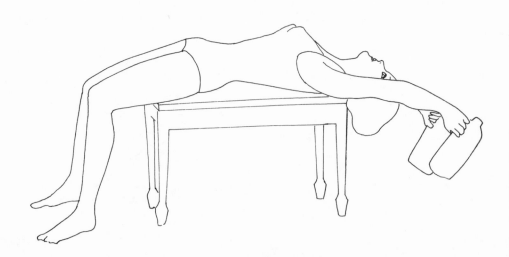

c. Flying Exercise with Dumbbells. Lying on the coffee table as for the Bench Press, lift the dumbbells at arm's length over your shoulders. Breathing *in,* lower the dumbbells, with arms almost but not quite straight, until they almost touch the floor to your left and right. Breathing *out,* bring them back to starting position. Do three sets of ten repetitions each.

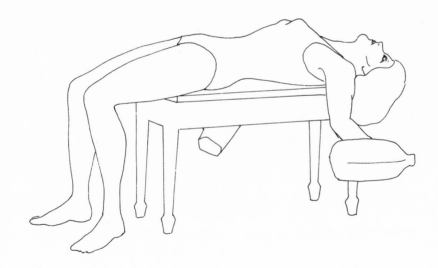

3. FRONT OF THIGHS

The Ankle-Lift. Drape your weighted bags around your ankles and secure them well. Sitting on a table high enough so that your feet don't touch the floor, and gripping the sides of the table with your hands, simply raise your lower legs until they're in line with your thighs. Be sure to straighten them completely. Lower your legs to the starting position and repeat.

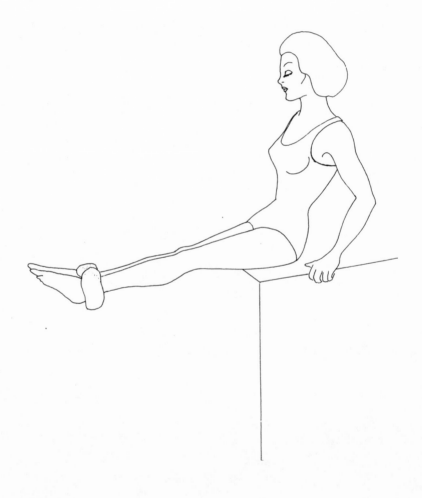

4. INSIDES OF THIGHS

The Split. Lying on your back, lift your legs, with the weights around the ankles, until they're at right angles to your body. Keeping your legs still at right-angles, spread them into a wide "split." Return to the starting position. Do three sets of ten repetitions each.

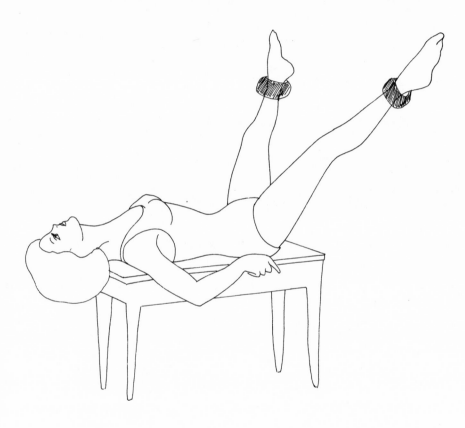

5. BACKS OF THIGHS

The Leg-Curl. Stand up, facing the back of a chair. Hold on to the chair as you slowly "curl" your leg upward toward your buttocks. Lower and repeat, three sets of ten repetitions with one leg, then do the same with the other leg. As this exercise becomes too easy, add another weighted bag to each of the bags around your ankles.

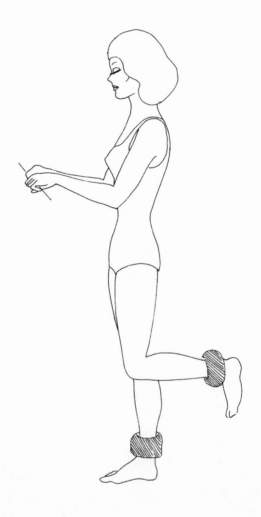

6. CALVES

The Heel-Raise. Stand with your toes on a doorstep, or on a very sturdy book. Holding on to a rail or back of chair for support, raise your heels until you're on tiptoes. Lower, repeat. Once three sets of ten repetitions become too easy, do the same exercise standing on one foot at a time. To further increase the resistance, hold a dumbbell in your free hand.

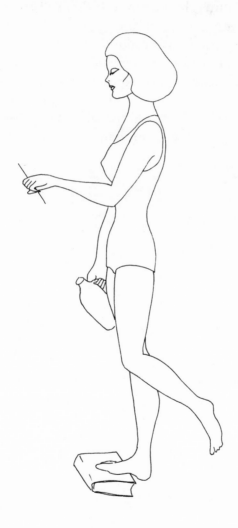

7. WHOLE BODY

The Squat. This is a terrific exercise for the legs and, done in a special way, also for the rib cage and chest. Stand up straight, holding the barbell across your shoulders. Take a deep breath. Keeping your lungs full and your back straight, lower your body until you're in the full knee-bend position. Immediately rise, pressing hard with your legs, and as you do so, exhale through your mouth. Repeat five times. On the sixth repetition, just before you go down, take three or four big breaths through your mouth. Hold the last breath as you go down, your chest fully expanded, exhale as you come up. Take three deep, chest-expanding breaths through your mouth . . . hold as you go down . . . exhale as you come up. Go on in this manner until the set is completed. Rest. Work up to three sets of ten, gradually.

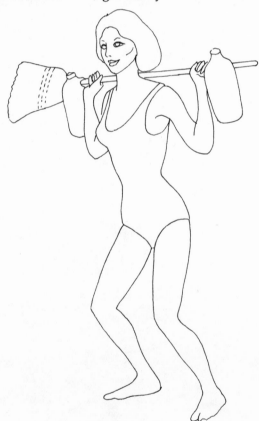

Continue taking your measurements every day, paying particular attention to the areas where you're building up your muscles. You want to reach your goals—no more. Unlike the male body builder who wants to have bigger and bigger muscles and more distinct definition, you want to fill out only to the points as indicated in your chart, then stop. So keep your eye on the tape measure, and on the mirror.

14

Controlling Your Energy Output

Before we go on to your marvelously satisfying maintenance diet, there's something else we must consider.

If we are to find your exact no-gain–no-loss equilibrium, food intake is not our only consideration: We must also be able to control your energy output. An extra 500 calories a day will not keep your weight steady if at the same time you're also undertaking some unaccustomed heavy sport such as playing an hour of squash every afternoon! On the other hand, if you become *less* active than you have been during Stage One of your Reshape course, even an additional 300 calories might put on more weight than you bargained for! So you must try to keep your everyday activities pretty much on the same level as they have been for the past few weeks. That doesn't mean that you cannot bring variety into your life—you simply have to *balance* your activities, just the same as you balance your calorie intake.

Let's start with the Reshape activities.

The in-bed exercises must remain unchanged—they're such an important beginning for your day! But during Stage Two of the Reshape Program you will be performing all the massage routines only once a week. The stretching exercises will remain, but the running-jumping-skipping routine will be cut to only three minutes per day. This will be balanced by the weight lifting, so we're back to where we were. As far as the Reshape activities are concerned, your total energy output will remain pretty much the same as it was during Stage One.

As for your normal daily routines, while you did not need to be concerned with them in Stage One (the more you did, the quicker you slimmed!), in Stage Two they must be under fairly strict control. For this purpose, the following Calorie Burning Table will serve as a guide.

	Calories per hour
LEISURELY ACTIVITIES (sitting, talking, sewing, dressing, sleeping, writing)	25-100
LIGHT WORK (Driving, dusting, mopping, office work)	100-200
MEDIUM WORK (Making beds, weeding, polishing, ironing)	200-300
HEAVY WORK (Shoveling snow, digging, sawing wood)	400-600

When it comes to physical exercise and to sports, the number of calories burned depends very much on the individual. As long as you remember that the range is from about 200 calories an hour for slow walking to about 1,300 calories for very hard rowing, you should be able to formulate a fairly accurate idea of your own calorie utilization. What matters is not that you should know exactly how many calories you're burning but that you should be able to balance each day in such a manner that the total for the day is pretty much the same as it was yesterday and as it is going to be tomorrow. If you played several hours of hard tennis yesterday, and you're going to keep it up three times a week for the next few months, then on the other four days of the week do some additional running to even the score. If, however, the extra energy output was just an exception, then simply allow yourself to take it very easy for the remainder of that day to bring about a balance, and take no further notice of it.

You don't need to become paranoid about it—even a substantial difference here and there will not matter too much as long as the *average* energy output over a period of one to two weeks is kept relatively steady.

15

The Stage-Two Diet

Our aim in Stage Two is to determine the calorie range that at your present level of activities will neither cause you to gain nor to lose, and further to pinpoint its uppermost limit.

In all probability you'll find that your no-gain–no-loss range is quite wide: perhaps between 1,100 and 1,600 calories per day. We must find the uppermost limit of that range, because that will be our starting point in Stage Three.

Add Calories Cautiously

Think of your daily calorie requirement, as you worked it out at the beginning of the Reshape Program, as your probable upper limit ("ideal" weight multiplied by 12 if you're under fifty, by 11 if you're over, plus 5 to 10 percent for extremely vigorous activity). Keeping your energy output as uniform as you can, cautiously add 200 calories to your daily diet for two whole weeks. If after the two-week period there's still a loss in weight and in measurements, add a further 200 calories and again continue with this increased diet for two weeks. When you reach a point where there's neither loss nor gain, very cautiously increase your daily calorie intake by just 100 calories for two to three weeks and continue in this manner until the arrow begins to nudge upward, or the tape measure shows a slight increase around hips, waist, buttocks, or thighs. When this happens, immediately drop *back* by 100 calories and stay at that level for a number of days, until you're quite sure that this is your uppermost no-gain–no-loss limit.

What You Should Add to Your Daily Diet

The additional calories should come from the protein and the fruit category. Do not add more fat, nor more cereal or starch, nor more vegetables. Keep the additions in the spirit of the Reshape Diet: wholesome, simple, natural, and nutritious. Eat an extra egg for breakfast, a one-ounce cube of cheese, a second serving of chicken or fish. Or instead of chicken or fish, use meat (use the calorie chart for protein foods on page 103 to guide you), with all visible fat removed. And for dessert, or as between-meal snacks, enjoy fresh, ripe fruits. Try to keep the additions in the same category each day, so that not only the actual calorie counts are unchanged from day to day, but also the type of food you eat. For this purpose, it is wise to write down each day exactly what you eat—this will help you plan your subsequent meals along the same lines.

Eat like a King!—or a Hearty Queen

You've been eating pretty well on a low, 800-calorie allowance. Just think how well you'll be eating from now on! Juicy steaks, rich stews, or whole small roast chickens alongside your creamy vegetable dishes! As long as for nutrition and *volume* you consume your two pounds of deliciously prepared fresh vegetables, you can probably eat as much meat and fruit desserts as you like and still be within your permitted stay-slim maintenance calorie allowance. So just go on; eat like a king—you'll never have a weight problem again!

Enjoy!

Now that you know the goals and the theories behind Stage Two of the Aussie Reshape Program, follow the simple Summary until you're satisfied that

1. You have positively identified the exact *upper limit* of your no-gain–no-loss dietary allowance and carried on for a number of weeks without change in your weight or measurements around problem areas.
2. You have corrected any posture faults you may have had.
3. You have built up shape in the form of muscles wherever needed (arms, chest, buttocks, thighs, calves), and you have strengthened your lungs and expanded your rib cage.

The catchword here is *enjoy!* Enjoy your great big satisfying meals . . . enjoy lifting your body out of a poor posture into a proud and at the same time relaxed carriage . . . enjoy building strength, shape, and good health through workout with weights.

See you in Stage Three.

Summary—

STAGE TWO

What You'll Need:

Broom
Small hard cushion
Pillows or blankets as in Stage One
Tape measure
2 empty half-gallon plastic bottles
2 plastic bags filled with beans
Slimming pants as in Stage One

You'll Do These Every Day:

In-Bed Exercises
(Details on page 65)

1. *The Stretch*
2. *The Vertical Leg-Lift*
3. *The Knees-to-Chest*
4. *The Scissors*
5. *The Isometric Ankle-Cross*
6. *The Isometric Wrist Push and Wrist Pull*

Stretching–Firming
(Details on page 71)

1. *The Reach for the Ceiling*
2. *The Side Twist*
3. *The Side Bend*
4. *The Backward and Forward Bend*

* *First Hard Call for Energy:* 10 jumps only
Rest, hips elevated, legs highest
* *Second Hard Call for Energy: Run, Skip and Jump for 3 minutes
only*
Bicycle in the air, then rest in
Antigravity Position

Posture-Correcting Exercises
(Details on page 135)

Check your posture faults. Do only those exercises which apply.

1. *Round-Shouldered Posture*
   a. Three-minute rest with small cushion under shoulder blades.
   b. Lie on floor, face down, hands behind back of your head. Raise head and chest, hold. Repeat.
2. *Slumping Posture*
   a. and b. as above
   c. On hands and knees, rock pelvis by lifting and sinking.
   d. On hands and knees, rock pelvis sideways.
   e. From standing position bend forward, hang loose. Uncurl spine slowly till erect, hold.
3. *Swayback*
   a. Lie on back, soles of feet flat on floor. Press lower back into floor, relax. Repeat.
   b. From standing position, drop forward, hang loose. Inhale as you contract abdomen. Exhale as you relax. Repeat. Uncurl till erect, hold.
4. *Knock-Knees and/or Flat Feet*
   Practice walking on the outer edges of your feet
5. *Bow-Legs and Outward Curving Ankles*
   Practice walking on the inner edges of your feet (on sand or on carpet)
6. *Turned-In Toes or Turned-Out Toes*
   Practice walking with exaggerated turn in the opposite direction.

Do These Every Second Day:
Building Muscles With Weights
(Details on page 142)

Check your underdeveloped areas. Do only those exercises which apply, three sets of ten.

1. *The Upper Arms*
   The Curl: use barbell. Start with hands at thigh level, palms facing forward.
2. *The Chest*
   a. The Bench Press: use barbell. Start at arms' length. Inhale as you lower barbell, exhale as you press up.
   b. Pullover: use dumbbells. Start with dumbbells by the sides, below bust. Inhale as you lift back, exhale as you return to starting position.
   c. Flying Exercise: use dumbbells. Start at arm's length as in Bench Press. Inhale as you lower dumbbells to the sides with arms not quite straight. Exhale as you return to starting position.
3. *The Front of Thighs*
   Lower-Leg Lift: use ankle weights. Sit on table, ankles together. Straighten legs to horizontal. Return.
4. *The Insides of Thighs*
   The Split: use ankle weights. Lie on back, raise legs, spread them wide.
5. *The Backs of Thighs*
   The Leg Curl: use ankle weights. Increase ankle weights as exercise becomes too easy.
6. *The Calves*
   The Heel Raise: stand on step or book. As exercise becomes too easy, hold a dumbbell in your free hand.
7. *The Whole Body*
   The Squat: use barbell. Weight on shoulders, inhale as you go down, exhale as you rise. For extra chest expansion, check details for full description.

DO THESE ONCE EVERY WEEK:

1. HAND MASSAGE (Details on page 77)
    a. Finger Pressure
    b. Massage of thighs, hips, buttocks
    c. 10 knee-bends

2. FLOOR MASSAGE (Details on page 79)
    a. The Side Roll
    b. The Side Rock
    c. The Fanny Press
    d. 10 bicycle kicks
    Rest, hips elevated, legs highest

3. FRICTION MASSAGE (Details on page 84)

4. THE SLIMMING PANTS (Details on page 84)
    While your Slimming Pants are working:
    a. The Wall Massage
    b. The Broom Handle Massage
    c. Run, skip, jump for 3 minutes only
    d. Bicycle in the air
    e. Let the blood flow back (antigravity position, or on cushions, hips elevated, legs highest)

Diet
(Details on pages 96-116)

Write Here Your Daily Stage-One Quota

FIRST TWO WEEKS:
Add 200 Calories (meat, fish, or poultry and fruit)

   If still losing weight,
NEXT TWO WEEKS:
Add 200 Calories (meat, fish, or poultry)

If weight and inches unchanged,

Add 100 Calories (fruit)

Watch closely for next two weeks.
When slight increase in weight and/or inches,

Drop 100 Calories (fruit)

Watch closely until absolutely certain.

Write Here Your Daily No-Gain–No-Loss Quota _____

PART IV

The Woman's Total Reshape Program—

STAGE THREE

FILL FAT CELLS FOR FABULOUS
FEMININE BUSTLINE; BLOCK OUT
FAT WHERE NOT WANTED, TO
KEEP NEW TERRIFIC SLIMNESS OF
HIPS, WAIST, AND THIGHS.

16

Breast Enlargement—How Much Weight Should You Gain?

Having worked so diligently to take unwanted weight off, you're probably panic-stricken at the thought of deliberately putting some of it back on again. Remember, though, rounding out your breasts will not only give you a fabulous bustline, but also balance your body fat in accordance with your body's requirements and prevent unwanted fat from creeping back to where you *don't* want it!

To put your mind completely at rest, let me point out that the actual weight-gain in breast enlargement is surprisingly minimal. Those among us who went from an A cup to a B cup, generally gained about one pound in overall weight. Those who went from a B cup to a C cup gained slightly more. But even those lucky ones who increased from an A cup to a C cup only gained about two pounds!

Visually, the changes were so substantial-looking that we just couldn't believe our eyes—or the scales—particularly since we realized that a little of that weight-gain must be distributed over other parts of the upper body as well. However, on checking with the manufacturers of the very lifelike breast replacement forms that women who've lost one breast wear inside their bra, we found that those synthetic forms, made to balance in looks *and in weight* the natural breast, only weigh a few ounces. The difference in weight between an A cup prosthesis for a size 30 bra and a C cup prosthesis for a size 36 bra is a mere 9½ ounces!

So go right on to Stage Three of the Aussie Reshape Program. You have absolutely nothing to lose, and all you'll gain is a better proportioned body with a terrific bustline.

17

The Stage-Three Activities

What You Do in the Mornings

One morning a week, you'll work out with your weights as you've been doing in Stage Two. This is to keep your newly shaped muscles firm and plump. Also once or twice a week, you'll slip on your slimming pants in order to get rid of unwanted fluid in the tissues. On a daily basis, your in-bed and stretching exercises are indispensable as always; they'll give a vital start to your day, and they'll keep your muscles firm and your joints and ligaments supple.

During this period of "building up," you must pay extra attention to your former problem areas with the various forms of massage you have learned, interspersed with "hard calls for energy"—however, since you do not want to *lose* more weight, these "calls" must be brief and not at all too strenuous. Two to three minutes of running in place and a few knee bends are all that is needed, and even these are to be broken up into one-minute segments. The purpose here is to make sure that if a few droplets of fat did manage to get through the various barricades, they will at once be dispersed and washed away— before they have time to settle in and harden into bulk fat. So use all the massage techniques you learned in Stage One—hand massage, floor massage, wall massage, broom-handle massage—and intersperse them with one-minute bursts of skipping, running, jumping, and with periods of rest in the antigravity position.

169

Massage of the Breasts

Our aim is to bring nutrient-rich blood to the tissues of the breasts by directing increased circulation to the area. In preparation for this, you will perform a gentle breast massage several times a day in the following manner:

Bend from the waist until your upper torso is horizontal. Cup your palms around your breasts and applying pressure with your palms, gently rotate the breasts thirty times. Still cupping the breasts in your palms, straighten up and gently pull them *up* and *out*. This technique will not only stimulate circulation, but it will also help to give your breasts a much more beautiful shape.

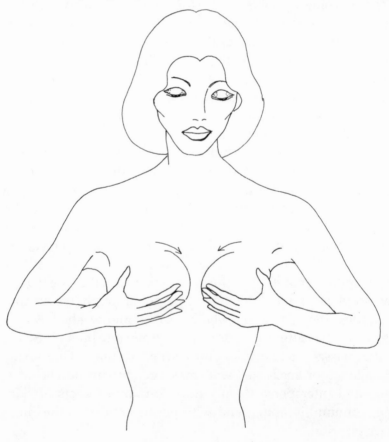

18

When Your Drink Goes to Your Chest

In Stage Three you don't need to drink more than two or three glasses of water. During this period, however, water drinking will have an additional, specific purpose.

You're already familiar with the effect of gravity on your body. In the case of fat accumulation, the process is slow and gradual; fluids, however, show up in the lower, gravity-prone areas within a very short time. If you drank a couple of glasses of water and then stood for any length of time on your feet, a "before" and "after" reading of the tape measure around thighs and ankles would show a very considerable difference.

Of course, in a healthy person such an effect would be merely temporary, so on the surface there seems to be no point in drinking glassfuls of water and then assuming the antigravity position: The fluids that will accumulate in the bust area will start trickling away as soon as you stand upright again. All the same, repeating the process two or three times a day seems very beneficial as a *preparation* for the actual breast-enlarging process: The unaccustomed volume of fluid seems to expand the tissues, making them more receptive to the nutrient-carrying fluids you will direct into the area later in the evening. So drink in the horizontal position as you've been doing during Stage One and Stage Two, then assume the antigravity position and rest for three or four minutes. You may actually feel a swelling sensation in your breasts.

171

Directing Blood Flow

While in the antigravity position, place your palms flat on the floor and press, tensing chest muscles as hard as you can. This will help to direct increased supplies of blood to the chest and bust areas. Do this a few times, then find the most comfortable arm and head position and breathing deeply, do some relaxed concentration.

Some researchers are teaching their patients to control their headaches by concentrating on directing increased blood flow to the hands, thereby diminishing the blood flow to the head. They report the hands actually becoming measurably warmer! We use the same technique for directing blood in the breast area.

Relaxed Concentration

Close your eyes. Take four or five deep breaths. With each breath, imagine yourself sinking deeper and deeper into something soft and fragrant and peaceful, such as a perfumed cloud or a mound of fresh rose petals. Concentrate on seeing the vivid colors, feeling the rich textures, smelling the fragrance. Now look inward into your body, and try to get a clear sense of your blood coursing through your veins, flowing down, down toward your breasts. *Feel* the blood filling the breasts, *see* them swell before your mind's eyes. Practice relaxed concentration while in the antigravity position, so that you will be able to use it effectively during actual breast enlargement later in the evening.

19

The Reshape Bra

A close-fitting bra, especially the lined or padded kind many of us not-so-well endowed ladies have felt compelled to wear, only serves to further flatten the chest. It compresses the tissues, hinders circulation, and in hot weather creates the type of "sweating-garment" conditions we've been using in Stage One to help us *reduce* by inches the natural padding on thighs, buttocks, and hips! Wearing no bra at all is better, but wearing the Reshape Bra is best.

"The moment I put on your unbelievable shaping bra," wrote Margaret from Perth, Western Australia, "I felt like a different woman. Instant uplift and inch-gain, and still the soft, natural, unfettered *me* underneath my clothes!"

The Reshape Bra is a very simple garment you can make in a few minutes from an old bra, or from a length of elastic and a bra-repair kit you can get at the lingerie counter of any department store. As you can see in the illustration, it simply lifts the breasts from underneath—just as when you're cupping them in the palms of your hands—enabling the blood to course freely through the whole area, feeding the tissues with its valuable nutrients. If you prefer a more covered-up look, you may add a piece of soft fabric, but make sure that it is loose and light and does not in any way press on the breasts or obstruct circulation. Wear the Reshape Bra as much as you like (you may even wear it to bed), adjusting it from time to time to make sure that the breasts are resting comfortably *on* the pads. Today's fashionable loose-fitting shirts and peasant blouses look positively voluptuous when worn over this foundation. And just think: While you're looking inches bigger with a soft, natural, braless feel and look, the Reshape Bra is actually at work developing your bosom!

What You'll Need to Make Your Reshape Bra

1. Length (approximately 20 inches) of 1¼-inch-wide elastic band.
2. Set of hooks and eyes from the bra-repair kit. Sew these onto the ends of the elastic band to reach firmly but comfortably around your chest, just under the bustline.
3. Pair of shoulder straps with the elastic about 20 inches long in *each* strap.
4. Two pieces of ½-inch-thick foam, 4 inches at its widest point by 9 inches long, shaped as in the illustration. If this is a little bigger than you need, cut around the pads until they fit.

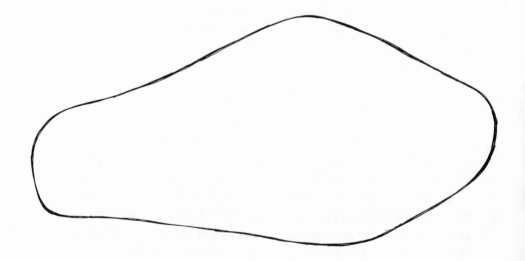

How to Assemble Your Reshape Bra

Fasten the elastic band around your chest, just under the bust. Attach the shoulder straps back and front. At the front, they should be stitched on just by the side of each breast. What you have now is the skeleton of an ordinary bra, without the cups. If you like, you can use an old bra, or buy a cheap one, and remove the cups. Be sure, though, that it is the kind that has the shoulder straps attached to the support band, not to the top of the cups.

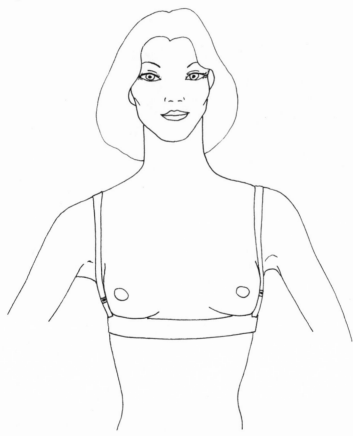

Place the pads as shown.* Play around with them until they're in the right position, held in place by the elastic band and the straps, protruding on top just enough to gently push up and support the breasts. Pin the pads in place, trim off whatever is showing *below* the elastic band, then take off the bra and secure the pads with a few stitches.

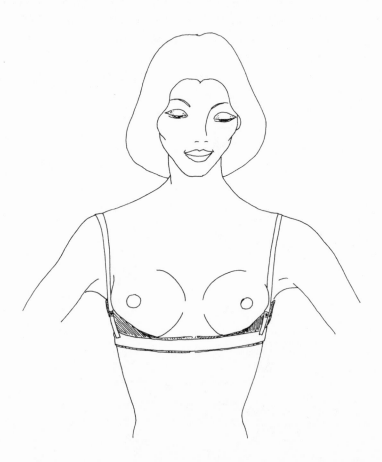

*The longer, narrower ends of the two pads meet in the middle.

20

The Stage-Three Diet

The Stage-Three Diet is precisely the same as in Stage Two: the no-gain–no-loss, balanced diet with one very notable difference: on days of breast enlargement, *you eat your lunch for breakfast and you eat your dinner for lunch!*

The reason for this unusual menu plan is that you must consume your no-gain–no-loss number of calories early in the day, so that by evening, when you undertake your actual breast-enlargement routine, your stomach should be empty and the nutrients of the day already well on the way of having been absorbed into the system.

Select your menus very carefully. Telescope breakfast and lunch into one meal, taking care that you consume the proportion of proteins, carbohydrates, and fats as you have been doing in the latter part of Stage Two. Your meal must contain the same number of calories—breakfast and lunch *combined*—contained in the earlier stage, and it must be of the simple, nutritious, and easy-to-digest quality to which you have become accustomed. Enjoy your next meal (your dinner menu) about four hours later. You should be finished with that meal no later than about 2 P.M. During the subsequent six to seven hours, you will have digested all of the first meal and most of the second. Some nutrients will still be in the process of being absorbed into the bloodstream; your blood sugar level will be normal (as will be the level of insulin), adequate to meet your metabolic needs.

It is at this point that you will introduce into your system a fast-absorbed, nutrient-rich drink and direct its course, as it is carried in the bloodstream, precisely to where you want its rich surplus nutrients to be converted to fat.

The Stage-Three Diet only applies to those days when you'll be actually doing your Breast-Enlargement Routine (that's whenever you have an hour of absolute privacy planned for the evening!); on other days, simply follow your normal no-gain-no-loss diet as you worked it out in Stage Two.

In case you're wondering what kind of meals you could serve yourself on the basis of breakfast and lunch combined, and dinner served at lunchtime, here's an example:

Let's suppose your no-gain–no-loss calorie allowance is 1,300 calories a day, or 500 calories over the basic 800-calorie allowance as in the meal plans in Stage One. Normally, the additional 500 calories could be distributed as follows:

BASIC BREAKFAST		1 egg	70	
		1 slice whole wheat bread	55	
		1 serving of fruit	50	
			175	
	Plus	1 glass skim milk	80	
		1 thin slice boiled ham	100	355
BASIC LUNCH		Vegetables	50	
		4 ounces ½ percent milkfat cottage cheese	90	
		½ tablespoon oil	60	
	Plus	1 ounce hard cheese	100	
		1 serving fruit	50	350
BASIC DINNER		3 ounces poultry or fish	120	
		Creamy vegetable *Gemüse*	255	
		Fruit	50	
			425	
	Plus	Extra serving meat or fish	120	
		Extra serving of fruit	50	595
			Total	1,300

On the mornings when you plan to do breast enlargement in the evening, make yourself a ham-and-cheese omelet taking 200 calories of cheese (2 slices) from the expanded lunch quota, and instead of 50-calorie strawberries, have a 100-calorie apple. Then serve your expanded dinner for lunch, adding a large green salad with oil dressing (the ingredients of the Hot Salad) to your meal.

21

The Magic Potion

No mysterious ingredients go into the miracle drink, for the secret of the Woman's Breast Development Technique lies not in the contents of the magic potion, but in the timing, and the conditions under which it is consumed.

You will need 2 ounces dried pears (unsulphured), ½ cup grape juice, and 1 tablespoon honey.

Soak the dried pears in the grape juice and honey until they're puffed up and the juice is almost entirely absorbed. Keep refrigerated until you're ready to use it in the evening, when you'll warm it by blending with hot water.

As you will remember, a sweet, warm liquid spends almost no time in the stomach (especially when the stomach is empty), but goes promptly into the small intestine, from whence it is absorbed through the walls of the small intestine directly into the bloodstream. By following radioactive glucose as it progresses through the body, scientists have been able to determine that glucose is capable of converting into fat in less than three minutes after entering the bloodstream.

Since your metabolic needs are being met from the nutrients you consumed during the day, and since your glycogen supplies in liver and muscles are kept at a satisfactory level and are not in need of replenishment, the newly introduced circa 300 calories will be converted into fat within a matter of minutes. Knowing *when* it will happen, you can quite easily control *where* this fat is going to be deposited—all you need to do is encourage circulation of the nutrient-rich blood into the bust area, while you hinder the entry of this fat-carrying blood into the problem areas of your body. For the next twenty to thirty minutes, all the tricks of the Woman's Reshape Program—gravity, constriction, heat, cold, muscle-tensing—will combine to help you achieve the realization of your dream.

22

The Breast-Enlargement Routine

Since your morning meal and your midday meal together have provided you with your whole day's calorie needs, all of the calories in your "magic potion" will be converted to fat. It will be your task in the space of about half an hour to an hour—the time, after drinking the "potion," that fat deposition of the newly consumed calories will take place—to promote fat deposition in the breasts while at the same time preventing fat from settling in your former problem areas.

As you will remember, "Fat tends to settle where circulation takes it . . . where there's room to settle . . . and where it can flourish undisturbed."

Conversely, fat is prevented from settling in areas toward which blood flow is temporarily obstructed . . . where deliberate constriction of the tissues leaves insufficient room . . . and where, if some fat does manage to get through, it will not be allowed to remain undisturbed.

Since by now you are perfectly familiar with the tools of the Reshape Program, and with their particular roles, the procedures that follow need no lengthy explanation. The only procedure that may need some clarifying is the use of *cold*.

In its efforts to keep interior temperatures at normal levels, the body responds to extremes in external temperatures by either dilating or contracting the tiny blood vessels that bring blood to the skin areas. *Heat* produces an immediate response of dilation resulting in *increased* blood flow to the affected areas; *cold* produces an immediate, intense vasoconstriction—a contracting of the tiny blood vessels, resulting in a severe decrease of blood flow. (At this point I must caution that this initial contracting of the blood vessels is followed, *after about five minutes*, by a vasodilation, in order to prevent tissue temperature dropping so low that it would cause frostbite. Because of this tendency to subsequent dilation of the blood vessels, we will not apply cold for longer than one or two minutes at a time.)

It is thanks to the above principle that a cold compress (or an ice bag, or a cold raw steak) succeeds in stopping the small subcutaneous bleeding that is the cause of a bruise or of a black eye: The touch of cold against the skin causes contraction of the blood vessels, preventing or restricting entry of blood to the injured area. And it is precisely this same principle we make use of to help prevent fat-rich blood from oozing in and unloading its unwanted cargo in tissues around the hips, buttocks, waist, and thighs.

(Here's something interesting to note: A recent newspaper report told of a brilliant new technique utilizing this same principle in the prevention of hair-loss in patients undergoing heavy drug therapy with a medication that as a side effect destroys hair roots in the scalp. According to the article, which claims a high success rate for the method, the patient's skull is packed in ice during the time the intravenously injected drug is coursing in the bloodstream, thereby preventing its dissemination into the scalp area!)

The Technique

Prepare the following, and place them next to your antigravity armchair:

Pantie girdle	fairly tight-fitting, with legs six inches long or longer.
Cream	a heavy cream such as lanolin, warmed in a dish of hot water.
Talcum powder	
Ice	Place ice cubes or crushed ice in each of two plastic bags (double thickness to prevent leaking). Tie at the top.
The "magic potion"	To prepare drink, place soaked pears and their juices in blender. Blend with hot water until smooth.

Take off your clothes. Apply warm cream to breasts. Leaning forward, gently massage the breasts with the palms of your hands, rotating them thirty times. Rest, then repeat.

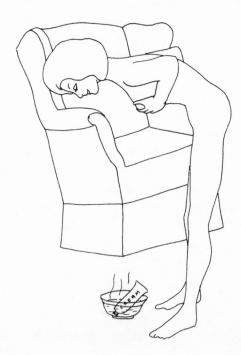

Taking one ice bag into each hand, very lightly stroke the skin only in your former problem areas: waist, hips, buttocks, thighs. Do *not* press the ice bags against the skin as this could cause "burning." Stroke quickly and lightly only until you feel a slight shiver in treated areas. NOT LONGER THAN TWO MINUTES.

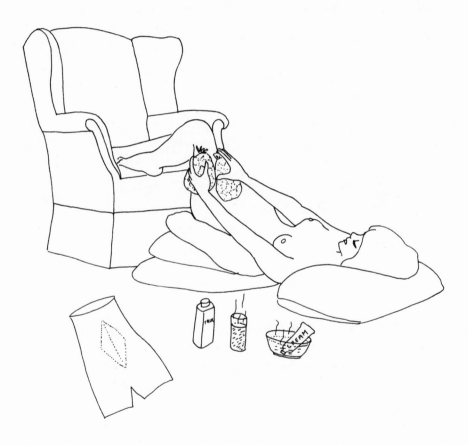

Quickly dust with talcum powder and slip into pantie girdle, making sure legs are pulled down and your skin is evenly compressed. Pass ice bags once again *over* pantie girdle. Slowly drink your warm magic drink.

When glass is empty, lie back on the floor. Elevate your legs to the seat of the armchair with your trunk horizontal on the floor; relax to a count of sixty seconds. Close your eyes, let your legs and hips become quite limp while you're counting.

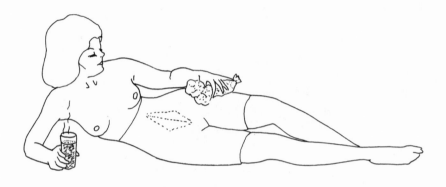

Slowly, without any jerky movements, assume antigravity position. From time to time, press your palms against the floor to direct increased circulation into the breast area. Do some relaxed concentration, looking inward into your body and *seeing* the rich red blood flow toward your breasts. *Feel* its warmth as it courses downward through your veins. *Sense* the breasts filling up and swelling out. Say over and over, "I can feel the rich, fat-laden blood flowing into my breasts." Then visualize the fat droplets settling in the tissues, beautifully rounding out your bustline.

Whenever you feel uncomfortable, lie on the floor, legs elevated, and gently massage the breasts with the warm cream, then stroke over the panty girdle with the ice bags. Keep

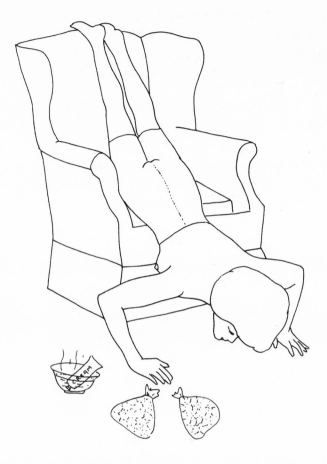

below-waist area *cold*, keep breast area *warm* and stimulated. Return to antigravity position. Continue alternating for about half an hour.

When thirty or forty minutes have passed, lie on the floor, remove pantie girdle, and stay in the horizontal position for a few minutes longer. Then raise your legs against the chair and gently massage the thighs and hips toward the heart. End the session by a minute or two in the back-stand position, hips supported on your hands, legs straight, toes pointing toward the ceiling.

Afterward, if possible, go straight to bed.

Try to schedule breast enlargement for consecutive nights—

five or six nights in a row for best results. Progress is gradual and it does no good to try to rush it by increasing the calories in your drink. If your body has too much sugar to deal with all at once, some of it might find its way into your former problem areas!

Keep your activities on an even keel during this period. Watch your calorie intake very carefully, consuming all your no-gain–no-loss calorie allowance in your morning and noon meals. And perform all the massages before breakfast every morning, ending each section with a spell in the antigravity position, especially on the mornings following the breast-enlargement routine.

You will begin to see results within a week or two. Continue until you're satisfied.

Summary—

STAGE THREE

What You'll Need:

Broom
Four pillows or one pillow and three folded blankets
Tape measure
Barbell or two empty one-half-gallon plastic bottles
Two bags of beans, 2 pounds each
Items for slimming pants
Small hard cushion

For breast enlargement:
Two plastic bags filled with ice
Talcum powder
Lanolin cream
Dish of hot water to warm cream
Pantie girdle, tight, with minimum 6-inch legs

For the magic drink:
Dried pears
Grape juice (no sugar or preservatives)
Honey

Do These Every Morning:
(Details on pages 64-92)

1. *In-Bed Exercises*
2. *Stretching and Firming*
3. *Finger Pressure*
4. *Thigh, Hip, And Buttocks Massage*
5. *Floor Massage*
6. *Wall Massage* (through your clothes)

7. *Broom-Handle Massage* (through your clothes)
   Intersperse with 1-minute runs, bicycle kicks and rest periods in the antigravity position
8. *Breast Massage* (Details on page 170)
   a. Rotate gently thirty times
   b. Pull breasts gently up and out
   Rest in antigravity position

Do These Once A Week:

1. *Your Posture-Correcting Exercises* (Details on pages 135-140)
2. *Your Muscle-Developing Exercises* (Details on pages 145-152)
3. *The Slimming Pants* (Details on page 84) *Important:* Skip, Run, and Jump for no longer than one minute.

On the Days of Breast Enlargement:
(Details on pages 171-179)

1. *Expanding Breast Tissue*
   a. Drink water slowly in horizontal position
   b. Assume antigravity position
   c. Press palms against floor to direct blood flow
2. *Diet*
   a. Shift lunch calories to breakfast
   b. Shift dinner calories to lunch
   c. Prepare Magic Potion

Breast-Enlargement Routine
(Details on pages 183-188)

1. Assemble by your antigravity armchair:
   • warmed cream
   • pantie girdle
   • talcum powder

- two ice bags
- sweet warm drink
2. Massage breasts with warm cream.
3. Stroke hip-thigh areas *lightly* with ice bags, *2 minutes only.*
4. Dust with talcum powder.
5. Slip on pantie girdle.
6. Lie on floor by armchair.
7. Slowly sip warm sweet drink.
8. Relax for 60 seconds while stroking through pantie girdle with ice bags.
9. Assume antigravity position, pressing palms against floor. Practice Relaxed Concentration.
10. Keep alternating numbers 2, 8, and 9 for thirty minutes (keep breast area warm, hip-thigh area cold; let blood flow to bust).
11. Remove panty girdle.
12. Lightly massage thighs, hips, buttocks (hips elevated, legs highest).
13. Stay in back-stand position (hands supporting hips, legs straight, pointing toward ceiling) 2 to 3 minutes.
14. If possible, go straight to bed.

How to Keep Your Fabulous New Figure Slim, Trim, and Shapely—Always

Diet You know your no-gain–no-loss calorie allowance. Follow it at all times, keeping your food intake nutritionally balanced, simple, and natural, and always basing it on a consumption of two pounds of vegetables daily, with at least one-half pound *raw*. Continue having three servings of protein foods (meat, poultry, or fish; cheese; and sometimes eggs) and at least three servings of fruit. The rest of your calorie allowance to be taken in one slice of whole wheat bread or some cereal, a bit of oil (or equivalent fat), a little flour for the recipes, and one or two tablespoons of cream or sour cream if you wish.

Continue weighing yourself *every morning* and do not wait for two or three pounds to creep up on you before you nip them in the bud! The moment the arrow nudges the slightest little bit over the uppermost limit (never mind if it's only retained fluid or whatever!), declare a semifast and have nothing but tomatoes sprinkled with your favorite herb that day, and a glass of skim milk with a teaspoonful of blackstrap molasses (you may sprinkle cinnamon on top for extra flavor) to promote peaceful sleep for the night. If you ever unavoidably overstep your uppermost no-gain–no-loss limit, do not wait for the extra calories to show up on the scales. Sometimes they don't show up for days! Just to be on the safe side, declare a semifast for the following day, whether your scales show any increase or not.

Exercise   No matter what your daily activities, do your in-bed routine faithfully every morning. Follow with three to five minutes of stretching-bending exercises and three to five minutes of running-skipping-jumping. Always finish with bicycling in the air, and a minute or two in the upside-down position.

Corrective Maintenance   Keep your eyes on your body; as soon as you notice the slightest sign, correct any faults that show a tendency to creep back. Do posture-correction exercises daily if you note some backsliding toward the round-shouldered, slumped, or swayback look. If the shapely muscles in your upper arms or thighs or chest show signs of shrinking, do three sets of ten weight-lift repetitions every other day for a week or two. If your tape measure or your mirror tells you that your thighs, hips, or buttocks have gained a fraction of an inch of fat, return to Stage One of the Reshape Program and do the whole bit—diet, massages, slimming pants—for a couple of days or so, until Reshape slimness is fully regained. Then follow with a couple of days on Stage Three to round out the breasts in case they've lost a little of their fullness.

Do stretching and bending or disco-dancing while you're alone, at your desk, or waiting for your favorite TV program to begin . . . walk briskly . . . breathe deeply in the outdoors or in front of an open window . . . find time at least once a day to close your eyes, breathe deeply and rhythmically, and relax, letting all your muscles go, and *thinking beautiful.*

Keep up these good habits for lasting youth and beauty as well as for good health. Ten, twenty, even forty years from now, you may still turn heads and win admiring glances!

Index